IS AIR POLLUTION
A SERIOUS THREAT
TO HEALTH?

Other books in the At Issue series:

Affirmative Action
Are Efforts to Reduce Terrorism Successful?
Are the World's Coral Reefs Threatened?
Club Drugs
Do Animals Have Rights?
Does the World Hate the United States?
Do Infectious Diseases Pose a Serious Threat?
Do Nuclear Weapons Pose a Serious Threat?
The Ethics of Capital Punishment
The Ethics of Euthanasia
The Ethics of Genetic Engineering
The Ethics of Human Cloning
Fast Food
Food Safety
Gay and Lesbian Families
Gay Marriage
Gene Therapy
How Can School Violence Be Prevented?
How Should America's Wilderness Be Managed?
How Should the United States Withdraw from Iraq?
Internet Piracy
Is America Helping Afghanistan?
Is Gun Ownership a Right?
Is North Korea a Global Threat?
Is Racism a Serious Problem?
The Israeli-Palestinian Conflict
Media Bias
The Peace Movement
Reproductive Technology
Sex Education
Should Juveniles Be Tried as Adults?
Teen Suicide
Treating the Mentally Ill
UFOs
What Energy Sources Should Be Pursued?
What Motivates Suicide Bombers?
Women in the Military

IS AIR POLLUTION A SERIOUS THREAT TO HEALTH?

Andrea C. Nakaya, *Book Editor*

Bruce Glassman, *Vice President*
Bonnie Szumski, *Publisher*
Helen Cothran, *Managing Editor*

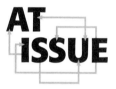
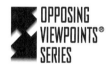

GREENHAVEN PRESS
An imprint of Thomson Gale, a part of The Thomson Corporation

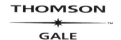

Detroit • New York • San Francisco • San Diego • New Haven, Conn.
Waterville, Maine • London • Munich

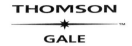

For more information, contact
Greenhaven Press
27500 Drake Rd.
Farmington Hills, MI 48331-3535
Or you can visit our Internet site at http://www.gale.com

LIBRARY OF CONGRESS CATALOGING-IN-PUBLICATION DATA

Is air pollution a serious threat to health? / Andrea C. Nakaya, book editor.
    p. cm. — (At issue)
Includes bibliographical references and index.
ISBN 0-7377-2392-0 (lib. : alk. paper) — ISBN 0-7377-2393-9 (pbk. : alk. paper)
    1. Air—Pollution—Health aspects. 2. Air—Pollution—Health aspects—United States. I. Nakaya, Andrea C., 1976– . II. At issue (San Diego, Calif.)
RA576.I686 2005
616.2—dc22   200440532

Printed in the United States of America

Contents

Page

Introduction   7

1. Air Pollution and Health: An Overview   11
   Pamela Myer et al.

2. Poor Air Quality Threatens Human Health   20
   Arthur L. Williams

3. Air Quality Has Improved   25
   U.S. Environmental Protection Agency

4. The Threat Posed by Pollution Has Been Exaggerated   33
   Joel Schwartz

5. Global Warming Caused by Air Pollution Will Harm Human Health   43
   Jonathan A. Patz and R. Sari Kovats

6. Global Warming Caused by Air Pollution Will Not Harm Human Health   49
   Thomas Gale Moore

7. Indoor Air Pollution Is a Major Risk to Public Health   56
   John Manuel

8. Air Pollution Is a Serious Health Risk in Asia   66
   Charles W. Petit

9. Pollution Regulation Reforms Will Worsen Air Quality   70
   John Edwards

10. Pollution Regulation Reforms Will Improve Air Quality   75
    Christopher Bond

11. A Global Approach to Pollution Regulation Is Necessary   78
    Christopher G. Reuther

Organizations to Contact   85

Bibliography   89

Index   92

Introduction

In October 1948 the small industrial town of Donora, Pennsylvania, experienced one of the worst cases of air pollution in the history of the United States. Sulfur dioxide, carbon dioxide, and metal dust descended from nearby zinc smelter smokestacks and were trapped by stagnant air. The result was a thick, poisonous cloud that blanketed the town for five days. At that time, most people were still unaware of the potentially deadly health effects of deadly air pollution; it was viewed mainly as a nuisance. So, although the residents of Donora could barely see through the smoggy air, they continued with their daily routines as much as possible, oblivious to the danger they were in. It was not until the smog lifted, leaving twenty-one people dead and six thousand people—a third of the town's population—sick or hospitalized, that many began to realize that air pollution was more than a nuisance.

The Donora catastrophe and similar incidents elsewhere during the mid–twentieth century changed the way many people thought about air pollution. As they began to see overwhelming evidence of the connection between air pollution and illness, Americans began to realize that poor air quality threatened their health and that, for their protection, emissions needed to be monitored and controlled. The result has been a succession of regulations designed to monitor and control air quality in the United States. Unfortunately, these regulations have been at the center of a heated debate between those concerned about human health and the environment and those in American industry.

In 1970 Congress passed the landmark Clean Air Act, which has formed the basis of the nation's efforts to control air pollution. The act gives the Environmental Protection Agency (EPA) the authority to establish and enforce National Ambient Air Quality Standards (NAAQS). The EPA monitors emissions of the six major air pollutants—ozone, particulate matter (such as dust, dirt, smoke, and soot), carbon monoxide, nitrogen oxides, sulfur, and lead. The Clean Air Act also charges the EPA with periodically reviewing the latest scientific studies regarding air pollution and reaffirming or modifying the standards as necessary to protect the public's health. The act was amended with more stringent emissions standards in 1977, 1990, and 1997.

As a result of the Clean Air Act, air quality has improved greatly in the United States since the 1970s. According to the EPA's 2003 air quality report, aggregate emissions of the six major pollutants have decreased 48 percent since 1970. This improvement has occurred despite a 42 percent increase in energy consumption and a 155 percent increase in vehicle miles traveled. Yet, according to the American Lung Association, in 2003 more than half the American population continued to breathe polluted air that was harmful to their health. In 2002 Bernie Fischlowitz-Roberts of the Earth Policy Institute found that the death toll from air pollution is high. He states:

In the United States, traffic fatalities total just over 40,000 per year, while air pollution claims 70,000 lives annually. U.S. air pollution deaths are equal to deaths from breast cancer and prostate cancer combined. This scourge of cities in industrial and developing countries alike threatens the health of billions of people. . . . While deaths from heart disease and respiratory illness from breathing polluted air may lack the drama of deaths from an automobile crash, with flashing lights and sirens, they are no less real.

There is sound evidence from hundreds of studies conducted worldwide that polluted air has adverse effects on health. Its effects range from mild respiratory irritation to lung cancer and cardiovascular disease. In developing nations, where air quality is frequently poor, the link between air pollution and health is often obvious. In China, the air quality in many cities is so bad that simply breathing is the same as smoking a pack of cigarettes a day, and respiratory diseases from air pollution are a leading cause of death. When asked to draw the sky, many Chinese children choose a gray or yellow crayon.

However, in the United States, where the sky is usually blue, and air quality has improved dramatically in recent years, the connection between air pollution and health is less clear. There is widespread debate over whether air quality is currently threatening the health of Americans. Some researchers are finding evidence of serious health problems from increasingly small pollution particles. In an August 2003 issue of *Science News*, Janet Raloff reviews the results of a number of air pollution studies, finding that "community death rates rise and fall nearly in lock-step with local changes of tiny dust particles—even when concentrations of those particles are just one-quarter of the federal limit for outdoor air." However, other researchers argue that there is no scientific evidence for such claims, and contend that air pollution is not a problem in the United States. Gregg Easterbrook, of the Brookings Institution, an organization devoted to research and analysis of public policy, states that the quality of U.S. air is so good that it should be "a national cause for celebration."

Disagreements about whether or not air pollution is currently threatening Americans' health fuels the debate over how air quality should be regulated. Emissions reductions can be extremely expensive for industry and, ultimately, the consumer. Regulatory agencies face the difficult task of weighing the potential health benefits of regulation against the costs to industry and finding the most desirable balance between the two.

Many people are critical of current regulations, claiming that the costs of the EPA's anti-pollution measures far outweigh the benefits. They argue that the huge expenses of implementing increasingly stringent standards impede technological innovation and hinder industry productivity, seriously harming the U.S. economy while only slightly benefiting the health of the American population. According to associate professor of economics Craig S. Marksen, in the Summer 2000 issue of the *Independent Review*,

> The Clean Air Act and its amendments force the EPA to mandate reduction of air pollution to levels that would have no adverse health effects on even the most sensitive person in

the population. The EPA relentlessly presses forward on its absurd quest, like a madman setting fire to his house in an insane determination to eliminate the last of the insects infesting it.

Critics of regulation charge that the EPA has squandered billions of dollars, with negligible results, and that the U.S. population would have experienced far greater benefits if this money were spent elsewhere.

Others contend that current regulation is not stringent enough. They maintain that human health is more important than industry profits and needs to be better protected. In a September 2003 statement, John Kirkwood, president and chief executive of the American Lung Association, states:

> Reams of scientific studies have shown conclusively that air pollution causes increased asthma attacks, emergency room visits, hospital admissions, and increased risk of death. A study conducted three years ago estimated that tens of thousands of Americans are dying prematurely each year because of our failure to clean up [industrial] facilities. Emerging research is linking pollution to lung cancer, birth defects, strokes and heart attacks. What is lacking is the commitment of the [Bush] administration to clean air and the health of Americans.

Proponents of stronger regulation argue that the development of new, cleaner technologies is usually less expensive than the prohibitive costs often claimed by industry.

In 2003 the debate over clean air regulation continued as the administration under President George W. Bush advocated controversial reforms to air pollution regulation. One significant change was to the New Source Review (NSR) provisions of the Clean Air Act. Under NSR, power plants built before 1977 must install modern pollution-control equipment when they expand or upgrade their facilities beyond routine maintenance. However, under a 2003 reform to the rules, some plants will be able to make modifications to their facilities without being subject to new emissions standards. The less-stringent rules also mean that the EPA will be forced to drop a number of current investigations of power plant violations of the Clean Air Act. The changes to NSR provoked heated debate from many different groups. Proponents of the reforms argue that it is possible to reduce emissions without hurting business, and that these amendments will allow industry the flexibility it needs to reduce pollution and contribute to a strong economy. Critics argue that the Bush administration favors industry over the environment, and that the modifications constitute a weakening of pollution regulation and will significantly increase air pollution.

Arguments such as these have been voiced since the beginning of emissions monitoring and regulation in the United States. Today there is still no uncontested strategy to clean the air to the satisfaction of health experts and environmentalists while easing the regulatory burden sufficiently in the eyes of industry. In the ongoing effort to balance the costs and benefits of regulation, there is continued disagreement over how to measure the value of human health and the value of economic growth, and how to create a regulatory balance that effectively protects them both. The authors in *At Issue: Is Air Pollution a Serious Threat to Health?* present various opinions on the effect of air pollution on health in the United States and around the world and debate ways to address pollution problems.

1

Air Pollution and Health: An Overview

Pamela Myer, David Mannino, David Homa, Luke Naeher, and Stephen Redd

Pamela Myer, David Mannino, David Homa, Luke Naeher, and Stephen Redd are epidemiologists with the National Center for Environmental Health at the Centers for Disease Control and Prevention in Atlanta, Georgia.

Pollution can be harmful to human health. Since the mid–nineteenth century, numerous organizations have been created to monitor and control outdoor air pollution—which is caused primarily by the burning of fossil fuels—in the United States and around the world. A succession of air quality regulations have also been enacted to protect human health. In addition to outdoor emissions from motor vehicles, power plants, and industry, potentially hazardous air pollutants exist indoors. They can often be detected through testing, and in most cases can be eliminated from buildings. While air quality in the United States has improved significantly since the 1950s, pollution still exists, and continual monitoring and pollution reduction efforts are essential.

W hether at work or play, indoors or out, we are all exposed to pollutants in the air we breathe. More work lies ahead to ensure clean air for all.

In the course of a day, we breathe 5,000 to 15,000 liters of air. With each breath, we inhale life-sustaining oxygen, which is absorbed in our lungs and carried throughout our body. Air also contains pollutants, including pollen, microbes, particles such as soot and dust, and gases such as carbon monoxide—substances that can harm the human body. Contact with these harmful substances, which are filtered through the lungs and can also irritate the eyes and skin, triggers several defense mechanisms such as coughing, sneezing, and the production of secretions. When these defense mechanisms are overwhelmed, human tissue is damaged or destroyed. Chronic or severe exposure may hasten the onset and progression of disease and even result in death.

Although air pollution has plagued crowded cities for centuries, several episodes in the United States and Europe since 1930 have driven home the harmful effects of air pollution. The worst air pollution episode in the United States occurred in Donora, Pennsylvania, on October 26, 1948, when sulfur dioxide, carbon monoxide, and metal dust emitted by local zinc smelter smokestacks was trapped by stagnant air and formed poisonous compounds over the industrial town. During the next five days, 43 percent of the 14,000 people in the community became sick. Ten percent of them were severely affected, and 19 people died. Statistically, only two deaths would have likely occurred in that small a population at the time.

Ozone is a powerful respiratory irritant that can interfere with the lungs' immunity, constrict airways, and increase respiratory symptoms in healthy adults and susceptible people.

Perhaps the most severe episode of ambient air pollution in the world occurred in London, England, in December 1952, when stagnant air trapped thick fog and air pollution for several days. More than 4,000 excess deaths were recorded. These acute episodes motivated the United States and other countries to implement ambient air-quality standards and strategies to reduce emissions that contribute to air pollution.

Since the implementation of these standards, air pollution levels have decreased in many parts of the world, but current ambient concentrations still cause adverse health effects. In particular, air pollution exacerbates chronic heart and lung disease and causes death. Although the most common cause of heart and lung illness and death in the United States is tobacco smoke, there is substantial evidence of the harmful effects of air pollution. One way to reduce our risk of illness from air pollution is to learn about the common air pollutants so we can control our exposure to them.

Outdoor air pollution

Outdoor air pollution is produced primarily by the burning of fossil fuels by motor vehicles, power plants, and industries. Concern about reduced visibility and evidence of adverse health effects led Congress to enact several laws concerning air quality. Beginning in 1955, air pollution research was authorized by the Air Pollution Control Act. Later, the 1963 Clean Air Act authorized the federal government to legislate and enforce air pollution controls. Paving the way for national air quality standards was the Motor Vehicle Air Pollution Act of 1965, which defined a process for implementing national emissions standards for new motor vehicles. But the 1970 Clean Air Act established the public health basis of the nation's effort to control air pollution.

Subsequently, Congress established the U.S. Environmental Protection Agency (EPA), and charged it with setting National Ambient Air Quality Standards (NAAQS) to protect the public's health, including the health of sensitive groups within the population. EPA's role is to identify air pollutants that are likely to endanger public health. Accordingly, EPA identified six air pollutants—known as the criteria pollutants—which pose the greatest threat to our health: ozone, sulfur dioxide, particulate matter, nitrogen dioxide, carbon monoxide, and lead. The Clean Air Act of 1990 also charges EPA with periodically reviewing and, if appropriate, revising the NAAQS to keep standards in line with current scientific knowledge.

After the United States phased out tetraethyl lead—a highly toxic additive that took the knock out of automotive engines—from gasoline in the mid-1970s to 1980, airborne lead levels decreased, and more importantly, blood lead levels among children in the nation also decreased. From 1988 through 1997, ambient lead concentrations decreased 67 percent. While lead from paint in older homes continues to pose a health threat, especially to young children, lead is no longer considered a major source of outdoor air pollution in this country.

Ozone. Ozone occurs naturally in the stratosphere, seven to 31 miles above the Earth, and protects human health by blocking the sun's harmful ultraviolet rays. In contrast, ground-level ozone is produced by chemical reactions with nitrogen dioxide and volatile organic compounds such as benzene and toluene in the atmosphere, and it is the main component of smog. Because the formation of ground level ozone is stimulated by sunlight and heat, ozone levels peak in late spring and summer and during the afternoon—when people spend more time outdoors.

Air pollution, once viewed as a local problem, especially in urban areas, has become a regional issue.

Ozone is a powerful respiratory irritant that can interfere with the lungs' immunity, constrict airways, and increase respiratory symptoms in healthy adults and susceptible people. Most vulnerable are the very young, whose lungs are immature; the elderly, whose lungs are less effective at filtering irritants; those with lung disease such as asthma and emphysema, and those with heart disease. While the adverse effects of short-term exposure to ozone are well documented, researchers are conducting studies of the long-term effects of repeated, intermittent exposures to ozone.

Particulate matter. Particulate matter includes naturally occurring dust and pollen as well as soot and aerosols from combustion activities such as agricultural burning, transportation, manufacturing, and power generation. The most harmful particles are not the large particles, which are mostly removed in the upper airways, but the small particles that may be deposited deep in the lungs. Before 1987, the standard for measuring particulate matter was based on total suspended particulate matter, no matter the size. In 1987, EPA changed its standard to measure only the percentage of particles with an aerodynamic diameter of 10 microns or less. However, recent research has shown that fine particulate matter—which includes particles with an aerodynamic diameter smaller than 2.5 micrometers—is inhaled deeper into lung tissue, and is therefore more harmful. In 1997, EPA issued new standards to address these smaller particles, which several epidemiological studies have linked with decreased lung function, increased respiratory symptoms, increased school absenteeism, increased respiratory hospital admissions, and increased mortality, especially from respiratory and cardiovascular failure.

In contrast to controlled laboratory studies, epidemiological studies measure human health effects of exposure to ambient air pollution. Ambient air typically contains several pollutants, and epidemiological studies allow researchers to evaluate the effects of individual and combined pollutants. Since epidemiological studies are observational, it is possible to study the health effects among vulnerable populations.

Indoor air pollutants probably have a greater impact on our health than outdoor air pollutants because people in the United States tend to spend more time indoors than outdoors.

Sulfur dioxide. The burning of sulfur, a natural contaminant of all fossil fuels, results in the formation of sulfur oxides. Sulfur dioxide is produced primarily by industrial and electrical power-generating processes involving fossil fuel combustion. Sulfur dioxide combines with atmospheric water, oxygen, and oxidants to create weak acids that fall to the Earth as dry particles, snow, fog, or rain, which is commonly referred to as acid rain. When these acidic substances fall to the Earth, they can harm vegetation and acidify lakes and streams. Sulfur dioxide can also constrict air passages, making breathing difficult for those with asthma, and may also alter the immune system and aggravate existing cardiovascular disease.

Nitrogen dioxide. Nitrogen dioxide is a product of high-temperature combustion and contributes to the formation of ozone. Motor vehicle emissions are the primary source of nitrogen dioxide in outdoor air, but power plants and fossil-fuel-burning industries also contribute. Nitrogen dioxide can irritate the lung and alter its defense mechanisms, thereby increasing a person's risk for respiratory infections.

Carbon monoxide. Carbon monoxide is produced during the incomplete combustion of carbon-containing materials, including gasoline, natural gas, oil, coal, wood, and tobacco. The principal source of carbon monoxide in outdoor air is motor vehicle emissions. Outdoor concentrations of carbon monoxide vary depending on how and where and when the gas is produced. For example, in urban areas, carbon monoxide levels are greatest in downtown areas where motor vehicle density is high, during peak commuting times, and in the passenger compartments of motor vehicles. Carbon monoxide interferes with the ability of the blood to carry oxygen to tissues; the most sensitive of these tissues are in the heart and brain. The health effects of carbon monoxide poisoning range from impaired mental alertness and performance, headaches, nausea, fatigue, and dizziness to coma and death.

Controlling outdoor air pollution

Strategies to reduce outdoor air pollution include implementing automobile emission standards, improving technology to reduce smokestack emissions of particulate matter, and requiring more-stringent standards for sulfur content in fossil fuels. Levels of the six criteria pollutants all decreased from 1988 to 1995. The greatest decrease was for lead, at 67 percent, and the least was for nitrogen dioxide, at 14 percent.

Air pollution, once viewed as a local problem, especially in urban areas, has become a regional issue. Sulfur dioxide, particulate matter, and the precursors of ground-level ozone can travel long distances. Industries contributed to the problem when they switched from short smokestacks to tall smokestacks, which released pollutants at higher levels in the atmosphere where they could be transported longer distances and cross geopolitical boundaries.

Several regional organizations have been created to address regional air pollution issues in the United States. These organizations vary in the composition of their members, but many include representatives from federal, state, and local agencies; environmental groups; industry; academic institutions; and private citizens.

The 1990 Clean Air Act Amendments, for example, established the Ozone Transport Commission and the Northeast Ozone Transport Region to address long-standing ozone problems in the northeastern United States. Commission representatives include governors and air pollution-control officials from each of the 12 members' states—Maine, New Hampshire, Vermont, Massachusetts, Rhode Island, Connecticut, New York, Pennsylvania, New Jersey, Delaware, Maryland, and Virginia—and the District of Columbia. Administrators from three northeastern EPA Regions also participate. To reduce regional air pollution, the members have agreed to introduce a low-emission vehicle program and to reduce emissions of nitrogen oxides.

Each year hundreds of people die from carbon monoxide poisoning in homes, automobiles, and other enclosed spaces with improper ventilation.

Aside from mandated organizations, there are also voluntary organizations whose mission is to find regional solutions to regional problems. For example, the Southern Appalachian Mountains Initiative, which is led by eight southern states in the Appalachian region, works with EPA, industries, federal agencies, academic institutions, environmental groups, and private citizens to seek solutions to the region's specific challenges. Because of the geography and meteorological conditions of the area, air pollution tends to stagnate over the area, which includes 10 of the nation's national parks and wilderness areas.

A larger regional group that works to address long-range transport of air pollution is the Ozone Transport Assessment Group (OTAG), which was formed to identify and recommend cost-effective control strategies for volatile organic compounds and nitrogen oxides to facilitate compliance with NAAQS for ozone. OTAG is a partnership between EPA and the Environmental Council of States and includes representatives from 37 states east of the Rocky Mountains, industry, and environmental groups.

In addition to regional groups within the United States, there are international agreements with Mexico and Canada to control air pollution. Created in 1994 under the North American Free Trade Agreement (NAFTA), the Commission for Environmental Cooperation addresses air pollution control in the three countries to ensure that pollution created in one country does not affect the health of citizens in another.

The creation of these regional and international cooperative groups is evidence of increased attention being paid to the necessity of addressing air quality issues across arbitrary boundaries. In addition, there is a growing consensus that a strict regulatory approach alone is inadequate to address these problems.

Indoor air pollution

While we've spent decades working to clean up the air we breathe outside, only recently have indoor sources of air pollution received much attention. Since the oil crisis of the 1970s, office and home construction of new buildings and retrofitting of old buildings have created airtight structures. In addition, new materials such as particle board and carpet can contain high levels of chemicals that are trapped inside and are emitted into the air long after installation.

In recent years, EPA and its Science Advisory Board ranked indoor air pollution among the top five environmental risks to public health. Indoor air pollutants probably have a greater impact on our health than outdoor pollutants because people in the United States tend to spend more time indoors than outdoors.

Tobacco smoke and emissions from unvented combustion appliances, woodstoves, and fireplaces are the principal indoor air pollutants; other potential pollutants include biologic agents such as bacteria and viruses, naturally occurring carcinogenic radon, dusts, and volatile organic compounds found in office and home furnishings.

Outdoor air pollutants may also enter a building through open windows or ventilation systems and contribute to the concentration of indoor air pollutants; the degree of infiltration depends on the characteristics of a building's construction and the efficiency of its heating, ventilation, and air conditioning system.

Moreover, while workers in factory and construction jobs are protected through the Occupational Safety and Health Administration from occupational hazards such as exposure to toxic emissions, no single federal agency has statutory jurisdiction over indoor air quality. The responsibility for indoor air quality research, policy, and monitoring is shared by several federal agencies. The EPA established a research program to address radon and other indoor pollutants; the Department of Housing and Urban Development sets standards for agency-funded projects and for mobile homes; the Consumer Product Safety Commission regulates injurious products that pollute indoor air, such as asbestos; and the Department of Energy has supported the development of more-efficient and less-polluting energy technologies, and it monitors the health effects of energy conservation.

Federal efforts to reduce indoor air pollution include developing voluntary industry codes, establishing product safety standards, publishing guidelines for dealing with radon, and offering guidance for handling asbestos in schools. Therefore, it is important for building supervisors in schools and office buildings, and individual homeowners, to educate themselves on the possible sources of indoor air pollution and to work toward reducing exposure to occupants.

Of the many possible sources of indoor air pollution, six pollutants are of particular concern in terms of public health.

Combustion by-products. Incomplete combustion of wood and fossil fuels such as coal, oil, and gas produces nitrogen oxides, carbon oxides, and particulate matter. The concentrations of combustion products in our homes depend on the efficiency of combustion and ventilation and on the maintenance and function of heat-generating equipment. Gas stoves, which produce nitrogen dioxide and carbon monoxide, are used by half of the U.S. population. The use of gas stoves for cooking in homes has been linked to an increased risk for lower respiratory illness among children. Gas or kerosene space heaters emit carbon monoxide, nitrogen dioxide, and particles, and these fuels contain high levels of sulfur. In addition, each year hundreds of people die from carbon monoxide poisoning in homes, automobiles, and other enclosed spaces with improper ventilation.

Tobacco smoke. Tobacco smoke contains more than 4,500 compounds, 50 of which are known or suspected carcinogens, and six of which are developmental or reproductive toxicants. The undeniable health effects of primary cigarette smoking include premature mortality, lung cancer, and obstructive lung diseases such as emphysema. Secondhand tobacco smoke, or environmental tobacco smoke, has been associated with low birth weight, sudden infant death syndrome, and acute lower respiratory tract infections among children. Secondhand smoke can also aggravate asthma, and it is associated with acute and chronic heart disease as well as mortality from heart disease.

Because of the considerable number of people still exposed to air pollution, we need continued evaluation of the safety of current standards.

Volatile organic compounds. Volatile organic compounds—gases that occur at normal temperatures from a wide variety of human made products—are emitted by modern furnishings, construction materials, and consumer products. One of the most common of these compounds is formaldehyde, which is used in many products commonly found in homes, such as cosmetics, toiletries, and the resins used in laminated wood products and particle board. Harmful vapors can be emitted for long periods after these materials are installed. For example, urea formaldehyde foam insulation, which became popular in the mid-1970s, emits a burst of formaldehyde immediately after application and then continuously emits lower levels. When improperly installed, formaldehyde can be released at high concentrations indoors. Formaldehyde irritates the respiratory tract and at high concentrations is toxic.

Asbestos. From the beginning of the century until the early 1970s when EPA banned its use in certain applications, asbestos was commonly used in building construction for thermal and acoustic insulation and fire protection. Asbestos causes lung diseases, especially a chronic irritation and inflammation of the lung, asbestosis, but also lung cancer and mesothe-lioma—a malignant tumor of the lining of the lung—among people exposed to asbestos in the workplace. Whether people in nonoccupational settings are at risk for lung cancer has not yet been resolved with certainty. Although asbestos use has declined in the United States, asbestos-containing materials are still present in many homes, schools, and offices.

Children . . . spend more time than adults engaged in vigorous activities, and therefore have a higher relative intake of pollutants into their lungs.

Radon. Radon is a radioactive gas created during the decay of radium, which itself is a decay product of naturally occurring uranium. Natural radon gas in the soil is the main source of radon in buildings and can penetrate through the foundation into the air in homes. EPA estimates that as many as 6 million homes throughout the country have elevated levels of radon. Elevated radon concentrations can cause lung cancer.

Biologic contaminants. Biologic contaminants, which are present to some extent in all buildings, can become airborne and enter our respiratory systems, causing infections and disease. They can also trigger allergic reactions and asthma attacks. Such contaminants include pollens; house dust mites; insect excreta and body parts; animal dander and excreta; and microbes such as viruses, bacteria, fungal spores, protozoans, and algae. Biologic contaminants can be found in any environment that provides nutrients and moisture for their growth.

Reducing indoor air pollution

The sources of indoor air pollutants are diverse and require different control measures. Control of environmental tobacco smoke, one of the most common and harmful indoor pollutants, can be accomplished by limiting areas where people can smoke. Employer and government policies have been successful in decreasing secondhand smoke in work sites and public areas, but these policies obviously cannot be enforced in private homes.

The presence of asbestos in a home or building does not necessarily indicate risk to health. Asbestos becomes harmful when it is damaged or disturbed and its fibers become airborne. Encapsulating asbestos by applying sealants to surfaces or removing it may reduce the risk of exposure.

Because radon can cause lung cancer, it is important to test for the presence of radon. Homeowners can purchase low-cost radon test kits or hire a trained contractor to test for radon. If high levels of radon are found, remediation may be necessary. This generally requires sealing a building's foundation to prevent soil gases from entering, or venting the gas produced underneath the foundation to the outside of the building.

Strategies for the control of indoor biologic contaminants include reducing relative humidity; repairing leaks and seepage from roofs and water pipes; properly maintaining heating, ventilating, and air conditioning equipment; and cleaning buildings regularly and avoiding the use of toxic cleaners.

Improving air quality for the future

Despite improvements in air quality, nearly one in five Americans, or 50 million people, lived in counties that exceeded the NAAQS for at least one pollutant in 1996. Because of the considerable number of people still exposed to air pollution, we need continued evaluation of the safety of current standards. We also need to incorporate new information into regulations to control air pollution, as EPA did in 1997 by recommending more-stringent standards for ozone and fine particulate matter, effectively doubling to 107 million the number of people living in polluted areas.

We also need support from the health community. A goal for reducing the public's exposure to harmful air [was] established as part of Healthy People 2000, a national prevention initiative. For two decades, the U.S. Department of Health and Human Services has used health promotion and disease prevention objectives to improve the health of the American people. . . .

Strides in improving air quality must continue, particularly to protect people most susceptible to the adverse effects of both indoor and outdoor air pollutants, such as children; the elderly; tobacco smokers; and people with pre-existing cardiopulmonary diseases, including asthma, allergic rhinitis, cystic fibrosis, and acquired immunodeficiency syndrome (AIDS).

Children, the largest susceptible group, spend more time than adults engaged in vigorous activities, and therefore have a higher relative intake of pollutants into their lungs. Children also spend more time outdoors than adults, particularly in the summer when ozone levels are highest.

Air pollution, whether indoors or outdoors, adversely affects human health. The effective control of air pollution will involve multiple approaches. Government can develop and enforce regulations to reduce ambient pollutants and environmental tobacco smoke, employers can encourage employees to carpool or use public transportation, and individuals can learn about air pollutants and make personal lifestyle changes to reduce their exposures. After all, improving air quality is everyone's responsibility.

2

Poor Air Quality Threatens Human Health

Arthur L. Williams

Arthur L. Williams is the director of the Air Pollution Control District of Jefferson County, Kentucky.

Since the implementation of the 1990 amendments to the Clean Air Act, there has been a significant reduction of air pollution in the United States; however, despite this reduction, poor air quality continues to be a serious public health hazard. Fine particulate matter poses the greatest health risk, causing respiratory and cardiovascular damage. In many U.S. counties, fine particulate levels continue to exceed health standards. Levels of ozone, another harmful air pollutant, also exceed health standards in many areas. Power plants and nonroad diesel engines are two of the biggest causes of particulate and ozone pollution, and until their emissions are reduced, air pollution will continue to be a serious threat. With hazardous air pollutants currently threatening the health of millions of Americans, further regulation and enforcement is vitally important for the protection of the population.

Editor's Note: The following viewpoint was excerpted from the testimony of Arthur L. Williams, director of the Air Pollution Control District of Jefferson County, Kentucky, before the House Energy and Commerce Committee, Subcommittee on Energy and Air Quality, June 5, 2002.

Notwithstanding [the] impressive progress associated with implementation of the [1990] Clean Air Act—progress that federal, state and local governments have achieved together —our nation continues to face air quality and public health challenges of substantial proportions. . . .

Perhaps the most complex air quality problem we face is achievement and maintenance of the health-based NAAQS [National Ambient Air Quality Standards] for particulate matter and ozone.

Arthur L. Williams, testimony before the House Energy and Commerce Committee, Subcommittee on Energy and Air Quality, Washington, DC, June 5, 2002.

Fine particulate matter and ozone

In 1997, EPA [Environmental Protection Agency] established a new standard for fine particulate matter ($PM_{2.5}$). Although [in 2002] we are still working to complete the data-gathering efforts necessary to determine which areas of the country violate the $PM_{2.5}$ standard, one thing is very clear: $PM_{2.5}$ poses the greatest health risk of any air pollutant, resulting in as many as 30,000 premature deaths each year. Additionally, fine particles are responsible for a variety of adverse health impacts, including aggravation of existing respiratory and cardiovascular disease, damage to lung tissue, impaired breathing and respiratory symptoms, irregular heart beat, heart attacks and lung cancer.

Fine particles are not only emitted into the atmosphere directly from combustion processes, they are also formed secondarily in the atmosphere from such precursor emissions as oxides of nitrogen (NO_x), SO_2 and ammonia; in addition to their adverse health consequences, fine particles also contribute to regional haze. Based on preliminary air quality monitoring data, it appears that $PM_{2.5}$ concentrations in 250 counties in the U.S.—located primarily in the East and in California—exceed the health-based standard.

Overall, progress in attaining clean air has been slowest with respect to ground-level ozone. In the southern and north central regions of the U.S., ozone levels have actually increased in the past 10 years, and in 29 national parks, ozone levels have risen by more than 4 percent. A significant factor in this trend is the increase we have experienced in NO_x emissions, which are not only a precursor to ozone, but also a contributor to such public health and welfare threats as acid rain, eutrophication of water bodies, regional haze and . . . secondary $PM_{2.5}$. Over the past 30 years or so, NO_x emission have increased by almost 20 percent, largely due to emissions from nonroad engines and power plants. Current data show that more than 300 counties measure exceedances of the eight-hour ozone standard.

In 1997, EPA revised the health-based standard for ozone by establishing an eight-hour standard, representing greater protection of public health. Litigation over both the new $PM_{2.5}$ standard and the revised ozone standard has delayed their implementation; however, the courts have now cleared the way for EPA, states and localities to move forward. . . . We urge timely and effective control programs for sources that contribute significantly to these air quality problems, including power plants and nonroad heavy-duty diesels.

Power plants

Electric utilities are one of the most significant sources of harmful air emissions in the U.S., responsible for 64 percent of annual SO_2 emissions, which contribute to acid rain and the formation of $PM_{2.5}$, and 26 percent of NO_x emissions.

In addition, electric utilities are responsible for 37 percent of U.S. carbon dioxide emissions and emit upwards of 67 hazardous air pollutants (HAPs)—including nickel, arsenic and dioxins—in substantial quantities. In fact, power plants are the major emitter of hydrochloric acid, which is the HAP emitted in the greatest quantity in the U.S, and are also responsible for more than one-third of anthropogenic memory emissions. The persistent and bioaccumulative nature of mercury makes it of particular concern relative to aquatic ecosystems, where it can contaminate aquatic life and pose a serious threat to humans who consume the contaminated species. Based on just such a threat, over 40 U.S. states and territories have issued fish consumption advisories for mercury for some or all water bodies in their jurisdictions.

One hundred and twenty one million people live in areas of the country that violate at least one of the six health-based NAAQS [National Ambient Air Quality Standards].

The magnitude of emissions from power plants, and the serious public health and welfare implications these emissions have, make controlling electric utilities a top priority. Fortunately, there are tremendous opportunities for doing so in a very cost-effective manner. Our nation's electricity generation infrastructure is aged, comprised of many 30-, 40- and 50-year-old plants that continue to operate without modern pollution control technology. . . .

Diesel engines

Nonroad heavy-duty diesel engines (HDDEs), including construction (e.g., bulldozers and excavators), industrial (e.g., portable generators, airport service equipment and forklifts) and agricultural (e.g., tractors, combines and irrigation pumps) equipment . . . are huge contributors to elevated levels of ozone and $PM_{2.5}$—representing a substantial and growing share of the emissions inventories for both NO_x and PM—thus posing a substantial threat to public health, including, among other things, premature mortality from exposure to $PM_{2.5}$. . . . In fact, the aggregate NO_x and PM emissions from nonroad HDDEs exceed those from all of the nation's highway diesel engines. In addition, the Clean Air Scientific Advisory Committee has concluded that diesel exhaust is a likely human carcinogen at environmental levels of exposure, further heightening the need to take swift and agressive action to control emissions from nonroad HDDEs. Given the limited authority states and localities have to regulate heavy-duty engines and their fuels, rigorous new federal standards for nonroad HDDEs and nonroad diesel fuel—equivalent to those for onroad HDDEs and fuels and in the same timeframes—are imperative. . . .

Unless emissions from nonroad HDDEs are sharply reduced, it is very likely that many areas of the country will be unable to attain and maintain national health-based air quality standards for ozone and PM. . . .

Hazardous air pollutants

The serious and pervasive public health threat posed nationwide by emissions of hazardous air pollutants (HAPs) is another continuing concern. . . .

Just last week, EPA released the results of its National-Scale Air Toxics Assessment (NATA), which provides nationwide estimates of exposure and health risks associated with 32 HAPs. According to EPA, more than 200 million people in the U.S. live in areas where the lifetime cancer risk from exposure to HAPs exceeds 1 in 100,000. Moreover, approximately 3 million face a lifetime cancer risk of 1 in 10,000. Considering that EPA has established 1 in 1,000,000 as the generally acceptable level of risk, these estimates not only illustrate the pervasive nature of the threat posed by HAPs, they also speak to the level of effort that will be required to reduce the risk and the high level of priority that should be placed on doing so.

According to EPA's data and information collected by state and local agencies, one of the primary sources of HAPs is motor vehicles, including cars and trucks. EPA has estimated that approximately 50 percent of all national HAP emissions, which do not include diesel exhaust, comes from mobile sources. The agency has further estimated that for more than 100 million people, the combined upper-bound lifetime cancer risk from mobile source air toxics exceeds 1 in 100,000. . . .

We must remember that the most valuable asset our nation can ever have is a healthy population and a clean environment. . . . Protecting these assets must be our highest priority.

With respect to industrial sources of toxic air pollution, the Clean Air Act called for EPA to establish technology-based standards for a large number of source categories by November 2000. These standards—known as MACT (Maximum Achievable Control Technology) standards—were to require new sources to apply state-of-the-art technology and existing sources to achieve reductions equal to those achieved by the top performing existing sources. Regrettably, EPA has not fulfilled its obligation; [in 2002] 36 MACT standards covering 62 source categories still have not been established. . . . Each day that these sources remain uncontrolled, many millions of people continue to be exposed to hazardous pollutants. EPA must do everything in its power to establish these standards as quickly as possible. . . .

Air pollution is a serious health threat

It is well established that air pollution presents a pervasive national threat to public health and the environment. The health risks are not only significant, we know of no other environmental problem presenting greater risk. Air quality regulators at all levels of government have worked diligently for many years in pursuit of our clean air goals. In spite of the considerable improvements that we have achieved, clean, healthful air nationwide still eludes us.

Over 160 million tons of pollution are still emitted into the air each year. One hundred and twenty one million people live in areas of the country that violate at least one of the six health-based NAAQS, not to mention the many millions of people who are exposed to toxic air pollutants that cause cancer and other health problems. The magnitude of our air quality problem and the associated health effects make it clear that funding for the control of air pollution should be a top priority. Unfortunately, the reality is that state and local air agencies are underfunded. Although states and localities devote significant resources to their air quality programs, air agencies have been operating for years with inadequate financial support from the federal government. As a result, many of our programs are not as robust as they need to be. . . .

Above all, we must remember that the most valuable asset our nation can ever have is a healthy population and a clean environment. In working to achieve our clean air goals, protecting these assets must be our highest priority.

3
Air Quality Has Improved

U.S. Environmental Protection Agency

The U.S. Environmental Protection Agency is the federal agency in charge of protecting the environment and controlling pollution.

In accordance with the 1990 Clean Air Act, the U.S. Environmental Protection Agency (EPA) monitors emissions and sets standards for air pollutants. EPA data show that from 1983 to 2000, concentrations of the six principle air pollutants—nitrogen dioxide, ozone, sulfur dioxide, particulate matter, carbon monoxide, and lead—all decreased. Levels of acid rain and other toxic air pollutants such as benzene also declined. As a result of the implementation of a number of air pollution prevention programs, air quality in the United States has improved significantly and will continue to improve in the future.

Under the Clean Air Act, EPA [Environmental Protection Agency] establishes air quality standards to protect public health, including the health of "sensitive" populations such as people with asthma, children, and older adults. EPA also sets limits to protect public welfare. This includes protecting ecosystems, including plants and animals, from harm, as well as protecting against decreased visibility and damage to crops, vegetation, and buildings.

EPA has set national air quality standards for six principal air pollutants (also called the criteria pollutants): nitrogen dioxide (NO_2), ozone (O_3), sulfur dioxide (SO_2), particulate matter (PM), carbon monoxide (CO), and lead (Pb). Four of these pollutants (CO, Pb, NO_2, and SO_2) are emitted directly from a variety of sources. Ozone is not directly emitted, but is formed when NO_x and volatile organic compounds (VOCs) react in the presence of sunlight. PM can be directly emitted, or it can be formed when emissions of nitrogen oxides (NO_x), sulfur oxides (SO_x), ammonia, organic compounds, and other gases react in the atmosphere.

Each year EPA looks at the levels of these pollutants in the air and the amounts of emissions from various sources to see how both have changed over time and to summarize the current status of air quality.

U.S. Environmental Protection Agency, *Latest Findings on National Air Quality: 2002 Status and Trends*, August 2003.

Reporting trends

Each year, air quality trends are created using measurements from monitors located across the country. . . . Air quality based on concentrations of the principal pollutants has improved nationally over the past 20 years (1983–2002).

EPA estimates nationwide emissions of ambient air pollutants and the pollutants they are formed from (their precursors). These estimates are based on actual monitored readings or engineering calculations of the amounts and types of pollutants emitted by vehicles, factories, and other sources. Emission estimates are based on many factors, including levels of industrial activity, technological developments, fuel consumption, vehicle miles traveled, and other activities that cause air pollution. . . .

The Clean Air Act

The Clean Air Act provides the principal framework for national, state, tribal, and local efforts to protect air quality. Improvements in air quality are the result of effective implementation of clean air laws and regulations, as well as efficient industrial technologies. Under the Clean Air Act, EPA has a number of responsibilities, including

• Conducting periodic reviews of the NAAQS [National Ambient Air Quality Standards] for the six principal pollutants that are considered harmful to public health and the environment.

• Ensuring that these air quality standards are met (in cooperation with the state, tribal, and local governments) through national standards and strategies to control air pollutant emissions from vehicles, factories, and other sources.

• Reducing emissions of SO_2 and NO_x that cause acid rain.

• Reducing air pollutants such as PM, SO_x, and NO_x, which can reduce visibility across large regional areas, including many of the nation's most treasured parks and wilderness areas.

• Ensuring that sources of toxic air pollutants that may cause cancer and other adverse human health and environmental effects are well controlled and that the risks to public health and the environment are substantially reduced.

• Limiting the use of chemicals that damage the stratospheric ozone layer in order to prevent increased levels of harmful ultraviolet radiation.

Nitrogen oxides

Nitrogen dioxide is a reddish brown, highly reactive gas that is formed in the ambient air through the oxidation of nitric oxide (NO). Nitrogen oxides (NO_x), the generic term for a group of highly reactive gases that contain nitrogen and oxygen in varying amounts, play a major role in the formation of ozone, PM, haze, and acid rain. While EPA tracks national emissions of NO_x, the national monitoring network measures ambient concentrations of NO_2 for comparison to national air quality standards. The major sources of man-made NO_x emissions are high-temperature combustion processes such as those that occur in automobiles and power plants. Home heaters and gas stoves can also produce substantial amounts of NO_2 in indoor settings. . . .

Since 1983, monitored levels of NO_2 have decreased 21 percent. These downward trends in national NO_2 levels are reflected in all regions of the country. Nationally, average NO_2 concentrations are well below the NAAQS and are currently at the lowest levels recorded [since 1983]. All areas of the country that once violated the NAAQS for NO_2 now meet that standard. [Since 1983] national emissions of NO_x have declined by almost 15 percent. . . . While overall NO_x emissions are declining, emissions from some sources such as nonroad engines have actually increased since 1983.These increases are of concern given the significant role NO_x emissions play in the formation of ground-level ozone (smog) as well as other environmental problems like acid rain and nitrogen loadings to waterbodies described above. In response, EPA has proposed regulations that will significantly control NO_x emissions from nonroad diesel engines. . . .

Ozone

Ozone is not emitted directly into the air but is formed by the reaction of VOCs and NO_x in the presence of heat and sunlight. Ground-level ozone forms readily in the atmosphere, usually during hot summer weather. VOCs are emitted from a variety of sources, including motor vehicles, chemical plants, refineries, factories, consumer and commercial products, and other industrial sources. NO_x is emitted from motor vehicles, power plants, and other sources of combustion. Changing weather patterns contribute to yearly differences in ozone concentrations from region to region. Ozone and the pollutants that form ozone also can be transported into an area from pollution sources found hundreds of miles upwind. . . .

Air quality based on concentrations of the principal pollutants has improved nationally over the past 20 years.

In 1997, EPA revised the NAAQS for ozone by setting an 8-hour standard at 0.08 ppm. [In 2003] EPA is tracking trends based on 1-hour and 8-hour data. [Since 1983], national ambient ozone levels decreased 22 percent based on 1-hour data and 14 percent based on 8-hour data. Between 1983 and 2002, emissions of VOCs (excluding wildfires and prescribed burning) decreased 40 percent. During that same time, emissions of NO_x decreased 15 percent. Additional NO_x reductions will be necessary before more substantial ozone air quality improvements are realized. For example, future emission reductions from existing and recently enacted NO_x control programs such as the NO_x SIP Call,Tier 2, Heavy Duty Diesel, Non-road Proposal, and, potentially, Clear Skies legislation will result in millions of fewer tons of NO_x emissions.

For the period 1983 to 2002, a downward national trend in 1-hour and 8-hour ozone levels occurred in most geographic areas in the country. The Northeast and Pacific Southwest exhibited the most substantial improvement for l-hour and 8-hour ozone levels. The Mid-Atlantic and North Central regions experienced minimal decreases in 8-hour ozone levels. In contrast, the Pacific Northwest region showed a slight increase in the 8-hour ozone over the period 1983 to 2002. For the 10-year period 1993–2002, the national trend in 8-hour ozone shows a 4 percent increase and the national trend in 1-hour ozone shows a 2 percent decrease. However, standard statistical tests show that these trends are not statistically significant. Ozone concentrations varied over this 10-year period from year to year but did not change overall. . . .

Although the recent national trends in 1-hour and 8-hour ozone are relatively unchanged, important regional decreases have occurred. EPA is continuing to investigate these regional assessments to further evaluate the trends in 1-hour and 8-hour ozone.

Sulfur dioxide

Sulfur dioxide belongs to the family of SO_x gases. These gases are formed when fuel containing sulfur (mainly coal and oil) is burned at power plants and during metal smelting and other industrial processes. Most SO_2 monitoring stations are located in urban areas. The highest monitored concentrations of SO_2 are recorded near large industrial facilities. Fuel combustion, largely from electricity generation, accounts for most of the total SO_2 emissions. . . .

Nationally, average SO_2 ambient concentrations have decreased 54 percent from 1983 to 2002 and 39 percent over the more recent 10-year period 1993 to 2002. SO_2 emissions decreased 33 percent from 1983 to 2002 and 31 percent from 1993 to 2002. Reductions in SO_2 concentrations and emissions since 1990 are due, in large part, to controls implemented under EPA's Acid Rain Program which began in 1995. In addition, in 2001 and 2002, energy consumption for electricity generation and industrial power leveled off; therefore, SO_2 and NO_x emissions from this sector did not increase as much as expected.

Particulate matter

Particulate matter is the general term used for a mixture of solid particles and liquid droplets found in the air. Some particles are large enough to be seen as dust or dirt. Others are so small they can be detected only with an electron microscope. $PM_{2.5}$ describes the "fine" particles that are less than or equal to 2.5 μm in diameter. "Coarse fraction" particles are greater than 2.5 μm, but less than or equal to 10 μm in diameter. PM_{10} refers to all particles less than or equal to 10 μm in diameter (about one-seventh the diameter of a human hair). PM can be emitted directly or formed in the atmosphere. "Primary" particles, such as dust from roads or black carbon (soot) from combustion sources, are emitted directly into the atmosphere.

"Secondary" particles are formed in the atmosphere from primary gaseous emissions. Examples include sulfates formed from SO_2 emissions from power plants and industrial facilities; nitrates formed from NO_x emissions from power plants, automobiles, and other combustion sources; and carbon formed from organic gas emissions from automobiles and industrial facilities. The chemical composition of particles depends on location, time of year, and weather. Generally, coarse PM is composed largely of primary particles and fine PM contains many more secondary particles. . . .

Between 1993 and 2002, average PM_{10} concentrations decreased 13 percent, while direct PM_{10} emissions decreased 22 percent.

Direct $PM_{2.5}$ emissions from man-made sources deceased 17 percent nationally between 1993 and 2002. . . .

$PM_{2.5}$ concentrations vary regionally. Based on the monitoring data, parts of California and many areas in the eastern United States have annual average $PM_{2.5}$ concentrations above the level of the annual $PM_{2.5}$ standard. With few exceptions, the rest of the country generally has annual average concentrations below the level of the annual $PM_{2.5}$ health standard. . . .

Carbon monoxide

Carbon monoxide is a colorless and odorless gas, formed when carbon in fuel is not burned completely. It is a component of motor vehicle exhaust, which contributes about 60 percent of all CO emissions nationwide. Nonroad vehicles account for the remaining CO emissions from transportation sources. High concentrations of CO generally occur in areas with heavy traffic congestion. In cities, as much as 95 percent of all CO emissions may come from automobile exhaust. Other sources of CO emissions include industrial processes, nontransportation fuel combustion, and natural sources such as wildfires. Peak CO concentrations typically occur during the colder months of the year when CO automotive emissions are greater and nighttime inversion conditions (where air pollutants are trapped near the ground beneath a layer of warm air) are more frequent. . . .

Nationally, the 2002 ambient average CO concentration is almost 65 percent lower than that for 1983 and is the lowest level recorded during the past 20 years.

Nationally, the 2002 ambient average CO concentration is almost 65 percent lower than that for 1983 and is the lowest level recorded during the past 20 years. CO emissions from transportation sources, the major contributor to ambient CO concentration, decreased dramatically during this period as indicated by EPA's improved new model of highway vehicle emissions. In particular, this report's higher estimate of CO emissions in the 1980s and early 1990s reflects an improved understanding of emissions from real-world driving. Between 1993 and 2002, ambient CO concentrations decreased 42 percent. Total CO emissions decreased 21 percent (excluding wildfires and prescribed burning) for the same period. This improvement in air quality occurred despite a 23 percent increase in vehicle miles traveled during the 10-year period.

Lead

In the past, automotive sources were the major contributor of lead emissions to the atmosphere. As a result of EPA's regulatory efforts to reduce the content of lead in gasoline, however, the contribution of air emissions of lead from the transportation sector, and particularly the automotive sector, has greatly declined over the past two decades. Today, industrial processes, primarily metals processing, are the major source of lead emissions to the atmosphere. The highest air concentrations of lead are usually found in the vicinity of smelters and battery manufacturers. . . .

Because of the phaseout of leaded gasoline, lead emissions and concentrations decreased sharply during the 1980s and early 1990s. The 2002 average air quality concentration for lead is 94 percent lower than in 1983. Emissions of lead decreased 93 percent over the 21-year period 1982–2002. These large reductions in long-term lead emissions from transportation sources have changed the nature of the ambient lead problem in the United States. Because industrial processes are now responsible for all violations of the lead NAAQS, the lead monitoring strategy currently focuses on emissions from these point sources. Today, the only violations of the lead NAAQS occur near large industrial sources such as lead smelters and battery manufacturers. Various enforcement and regulatory actions are being actively pursued by EPA and the states for cleaning up these sources.

Acid rain

Acidic deposition or "acid rain" occurs when emissions of sulfur dioxide and nitrogen oxides in the atmosphere react with water, oxygen, and oxidants to form acidic compounds. These compounds fall to the Earth in either dry form (gas and particles) or wet form (rain, snow, and fog). Some are carried by the wind, sometimes hundreds of miles, across state and national borders. In the United States, about 63 percent of annual SO_2 emissions and 22 percent of NO_x emissions are produced by burning fossil fuels for electricity generation. . . .

SO_2 emissions reductions were significant in the first 6 years of EPA's Acid Rain Program. In 2002, sources in the Acid Rain Program emitted 10.2 million tons, down from 15.7 million tons in 1990. Emissions of SO_2 in 2002 were 400,000 tons less than in 2001. . . .

NO_x emissions from all Acid Rain Program sources have also declined since 1990. NO_x emissions have decreased steadily from 6 million tons in 1997 to 4.5 million tons in 2002. The more than 1,000 sources affected by the Acid Rain NO_x Program emitted 4.1 million tons in 2000, approximately 1.5 million tons (25 percent) less than they did in 1990. NO_x emissions from these sources in 2001 were 3.6 million tons (over 40 percent) below what emissions were projected to have been in 2000 without the Acid Rain Program.

Toxic air pollutants

Toxic air pollutants, or air toxics, are those pollutants that cause or may cause cancer or other serious health effects, such as reproductive effects or birth defects. Air toxics may also cause adverse environmental and ecological effects. Examples of toxic air pollutants include benzene, found in gasoline; perchloroethylene, emitted from some dry cleaning facilities; and methylene chloride, used as a solvent by a number of industries. Most air toxics originate from man-made sources, including mobile sources (e.g., cars, trucks, construction equipment) and stationary sources (e.g., factories, refineries, power plants), as well as indoor sources (e.g., some building materials and cleaning solvents). Some air toxics are also released from natural sources such as volcanic eruptions and forest fires. The Clean Air Act identifies 188 air toxics from industrial sources. EPA has identified 21 pollutants as mobile source air toxics, including diesel particulate matter and diesel exhaust organic gases. In addition, EPA has listed 33 urban hazardous air pollutants that pose the greatest threats to public health in urban areas. . . .

EPA and state regulations, as well as voluntary reductions by industry, have clearly achieved large reductions in overall air toxic emissions.

Based on the data in the NEI [National Emissions Inventory], estimates of nationwide air toxics emissions decreased by approximately 24 percent between baseline (1990–1993) and 1996. Thirty-three of these air toxics that pose the greatest threat to public health in urban areas have similarly decreased 31 percent. Although changes in how EPA compiled the national inventory over time may account for some differences, EPA and state regulations, as well as voluntary reductions by industry, have clearly achieved large reductions in overall air toxic emissions.

Trends for individual air toxics vary from pollutant to pollutant. Benzene, which is the most widely monitored toxic air pollutant, is emitted from cars, trucks, oil refineries, and chemical processes. The graph below shows trends for benzene at 95 urban monitoring sites around the country. These urban areas generally have higher levels of benzene than other areas of the country. Measurements taken at these sites show, on average, a 47 percent drop in benzene levels from 1994 to 2000. During this period, EPA phased in new (so-called tier 1) car emission standards; required many cities to begin using cleaner burning gasoline; and set standards that required significant reductions in benzene and other pollutants emitted from oil refineries and chemical processes. EPA estimates that benzene emissions from all sources dropped 20 percent nationwide from 1990 to 1996. . . .

Programs to reduce air toxics

Since 1990, EPA's technology-based emission standards for industrial and combustion sources (e.g., chemical plants, oil refineries, dry cleaners, and municipal waste combustors) have proven extremely successful in reducing emissions of air toxics. Once fully implemented, these standards will cut annual emissions of toxic air pollutants by nearly 1.5 million tons from 1990 levels. Of this total reduction, dioxin emissions from municipal waste combustors and municipal waste incinerator units will have been reduced by approximately 99 percent and mercury emissions by 95 percent. Additional reductions are expected by 2005. EPA has also put into place important controls for motor vehicles and their fuels, including introduction of reformulated gasoline and low sulfur diesel fuel, and is taking additional steps to reduce air toxics from vehicles. Furthermore, air toxics emissions will further decline as the motor vehicle fleet turns over, with newer vehicles replacing older higher-emitting vehicles. By the year 2020, these requirements are expected to reduce emissions of a number of air toxics (benzene, formaldehyde, acetaldehyde, and 1,3-butadiene) from highway motor vehicles by about 75 percent and diesel PM by over 90 percent from 1990 levels. . . .

Improvements

The Clean Air Act has resulted in many improvements in the quality of the air in the United States. Scientific and international developments continue to have an effect on the air pollution programs that are implemented by the U.S. Environmental Protection Agency and state, local, and tribal agencies. New data help identify sources of pollutants and the properties of these pollutants. Although much progress has been made to clean up our air, work must continue to ensure steady improvements in air quality, especially because our lifestyles create more pollution sources. Many of the strategies for air quality improvement will continue to be developed through coordinated efforts with EPA, state, local, and tribal governments, as well as industry and other environmental organizations.

4

The Threat Posed by Pollution Has Been Exaggerated

Joel Schwartz

Joel Schwartz is a senior fellow in the Environment Program at the Reason Public Policy Institute, a public-policy think tank that promotes market competition. He has written numerous articles on the links between air pollution and health.

Air pollution has been substantially reduced in the United States over the past few decades, yet a majority of Americans falsely believe that air quality has worsened and seriously threatens their health. This belief is due to misleading reports by environmentalists and regulatory agencies. The American Lung Association, the Public Interest Research Group, and the Environmental Protection Agency have all exaggerated the frequency and geographic extent of harmful ozone levels, and often blur the distinction between modest and severe health risks associated with air pollution. The data show that ozone levels have actually declined, despite an increase in population and vehicle travel, and will continue to decline in the future.

The United States has made dramatic progress in reducing air pollution over the last few decades, and most American cities now enjoy relatively good air quality. But polls show that most Americans believe air pollution has grown worse or will become worse in the future, and that most people face serious risks from air pollution.

This disconnect between perception and reality is, in part, the result of environmental activists' exaggerations of air pollution levels and risks, which make air pollution appear to be increasing when in fact it has been declining. State and federal regulatory agencies sometimes also resort to such tactics, and the media generally report those claims uncritically. As a result, public fears over air pollution are out of all proportion to the actual risks posed by current air pollution levels, and there is widespread but unwarranted pessimism about the nation's prospects for further air pollution improvements.

If people overestimate their exposure to and risk from air pollution, they will demand stricter, more costly air pollution regulation. We face many threats to our health and safety, but have limited resources with which to address them: by devoting excessive resources to one exaggerated risk, we are less able to counter other genuinely more serious risks. People can make informed decisions about air pollution control only if they have accurate information on the risks they face.

Perception and reality

The Environmental Protection Agency (EPA) monitors ozone and other air pollutants at hundreds of locations around the United States. EPA has two ozone standards: The first, known as the "one-hour standard," requires that daily ozone levels exceed 125 parts per billion (ppb) on no more than three days in any consecutive three-year period. Ozone levels are determined based on hourly averages (hence the name of the standard). EPA's "eight-hour standard," promulgated in 1997 is more stringent. It requires that the average of the fourth-highest daily, eight-hour average ozone level from each of the most recent three years not exceed 85 ppb. The standards are difficult to compare because of their different forms, but the one-hour standard is roughly equivalent to an eight-hour standard set at about 95 ppb.

In the early 1980s, half of the nation's monitoring stations registered ozone in excess of the federal one-hour health standard, and they averaged more than 12 such exceedances per year. But as of the end of 2002, only 13 percent of the stations failed the one-hour standard and they averaged just four exceedances per year. . . . Even the most polluted areas of the country achieved impressive ozone reductions during the last 20 years. About 40 percent of monitoring locations currently exceed the more stringent eight-hour standard, but peak eight-hour ozone levels are also declining in most areas.

Public fears over air pollution are out of all proportion to the actual risks posed by current air pollution levels.

The nation's success with air quality extends beyond ozone to other pollutants. For example, between 1981 and 2000, carbon monoxide (CO) declined 61 percent, sulfur dioxide (SO_2) 50 percent, and nitrogen oxides (NO_x) 14 percent. Only two among hundreds of the nation's monitoring locations still exceed the CO and SO_2 standards. All areas of the country meet the NO_x standard. For all three pollutants, pollution levels are well below the EPA standards in almost all cases.

Likewise, airborne particulate matter (PM) has also registered large declines. $PM_{2.5}$ (PM up to 2.5 microns in diameter) dropped 33 percent from 1980 to 2000, while the soot emissions rate from diesel trucks is down almost 85 percent since 1975.

This downward trend in pollution levels will continue. On-road pollution measurements show per-mile emissions from gasoline vehicles are dropping by about 10 percent per year as the fleet turns over to more recent models that start out and stay much cleaner than vehicles built years ago. Diesel truck emissions are also declining, albeit about half as fast. Although motorists are driving more miles each year and population growth means more motorists on the roads, the increases in driving are tiny compared to the large declines in vehicle emission rates and will do little to slow progress on auto pollution.

Emissions from industrial sources will also continue to drop. Starting in 2004, EPA regulations require a 60 percent reduction in warm-season NO_x emissions from coal-fired power plants and industrial boilers—the major industrial sources of ozone-forming pollution. The federal Clean Air Act requires a 20 percent reduction in PM-forming SO_2 from power plants between 2000 and 2010. Those reductions are in addition to substantial declines in industrial NO_x and SO_2 emissions over the last 30 years.

Misperceptions

Despite past success in reducing air pollution and the positive outlook for the future, polls show most Americans think air pollution is getting worse. For example:

• A January 2002 Wirthlin Poll found that 66 percent of Americans believe air pollution has gotten worse during the past 10 years, up from 61 percent two years before, while a poll commissioned by Environmental Defense in 2000 found that 57 percent of Americans believe environmental conditions have gotten worse during the last 30 years.

• Americans also believe that environmental quality will decline in the future. The 2000 Environmental Defense poll found that 67 percent of Americans believe air pollution will continue to get worse. Likewise, a March 2001 Gallup Poll found that 57 percent of Americans believe environmental quality is deteriorating. A 1999 *Washington Post* poll found that 51 percent of Americans believe pollution will greatly increase in the future, up from 44 percent in 1996. State-based surveys have found similar results. The Public Policy Institute of California recently reported that 78 percent of Californians believe the state has made only "some" or "hardly any" progress in solving environmental problems.

• Most Americans also believe air pollution is still a serious threat to their health. Some 80 percent of New Yorkers rate air pollution as a "very serious" or "somewhat serious" problem, as do 77 percent of Texans. When asked about the most serious environmental issue facing California, a 34 percent plurality chose air pollution, with "growth" coming in a distant second at 13 percent.

According to the old saying, "It's not the things we didn't know that hurt us; it's the things we knew for sure that turned out to be wrong." When it comes to air pollution, why do most Americans "know" so much that is not so? Americans consider environmental groups the most credible sources of information on the environment, yet those activist groups consistently provide misleading information on air pollution levels, trends, risks, and prospects. Americans also trust information from regulatory agencies, yet the agencies often paint a misleadingly pessimistic picture. At the same time, the media often provide extensive coverage of air pollution reports and press releases from environmentalists and government regulators, yet the press reports rarely include critical examination or context on the claims those organizations make.

Inflating air pollution exposure

In its report "State of the Air 2003," the American Lung Association claimed that between 1999 and 2001, Los Angeles County averaged 35 days per year with ozone in excess of EPA's eighth-our ozone benchmark of 85 ppb. Yet . . . none of L.A. County's 14 ozone monitors registered anywhere near that many ozone exceedances. Indeed, the average L.A. County location averaged six exceedances per year—83 percent less than the report claims—while the most densely populated areas of the county never exceeded the EPA benchmark at all.

The American Lung Association derived its inflated value by assigning an ozone violation to the entire county on any day in which at least one location in the county exceeded 85 ppb. For example, if ozone was high one day in Glendora and the next day in Santa Clarita, 50 miles away, the report counted two high-ozone days for all 9.5 million people in L.A. County. The logical fallacy here is obvious—it is like failing an entire class when one student does poorly.

The American Lung Association method exaggerates ozone exposure for tens of millions of people all across the country. . . . For each county, the dash at the top marks the report's artificially inflated claim, while the other markers show the actual number of elevated ozone days per year at the worst, average, and best location in each county, reading from top to bottom. The average location in a county typically has less than half as many ozone exceedances as the report claims for the entire county.

> *Americans consider environmental groups the most credible sources of information on the environment, yet those activist groups consistently provide misleading information.*

The Public Interest Research Group (PIRG) took the American Lung Association's techniques to the state level. In its 2002 report "Danger in the Air," PIRG claimed that California exceeded the eight-hour ozone benchmark on 130 days in 2001. Yet almost half of the state's monitoring locations had no exceedances, while the average location had seven. Even the worst location in California had only about half as many ozone exceedances as PIRG claimed for the whole state. PIRG similarly claimed fictionally large ozone problems for every other state it scrutinized.

Regulatory agencies often take a similar tack in reporting ozone levels. For example, EPA recently downgraded California's San Joaquin Valley air district—a multi-county region—from "serious" to "severe" for the one-hour ozone standard. The change gave the region more time to attain the standard, but also required more stringent air pollution controls. In its press release on the action, EPA stated, "Air quality data from 1997 through 1999 indicates the San Joaquin Valley experienced 80 days of unhealthy levels of ozone air pollution." Yet Clovis, a suburb of Fresno and the most polluted location in the valley, had 40 days above the one-hour benchmark, while nearly half of the valley's monitoring locations actually complied with the one-hour ozone standard.

One might argue that talking about the number of days smog is elevated somewhere in a region is not misleading and paints a fair picture of the nature of the regional pollution problem. But the health effects of smog depend on how often a given person is exposed. Because no one is exposed to smog anywhere near as often as the activists' reports claim, the public is being encouraged to vastly overestimate its risk from air pollution.

Though dozens of newspapers covered one or more of those reports, most did not include any critical analysis of the proponents' assertions. Only about one in 10 papers flagged concerns regarding the fictional ozone exposure claims.

How widespread is air pollution?

In the latest installment of its annual air pollution trends report, EPA claimed that 133 million Americans breathe air that exceeds one or more federal air pollution standards—mainly the tough new annual $PM_{2.5}$ and eight-hour ozone standards. Yet EPA's claim is a substantial exaggeration.

The agency classifies Clean Air Act compliance status at the county level. For example, if any air pollution monitor in a county registers ozone in excess of federal requirements, that county is classified as "nonattainment." Regional classification often makes sense because pollution can be transported many miles from its source. The problem arises because EPA also uses county non-attainment status when counting the number of people who breathe polluted air. Because only one location in a county need exceed an air standard for the entire county to be classified as nonattainment, many people in a non-attainment county might still breathe clean air. Indeed, this situation is the norm, rather than the exception. . . .

Most counties have at least some areas with clean air based on the federal standards. For some counties, the vast majority of locations have clean air based on either standard. The percentage of people breathing clean air is also often greater than the monitoring data suggest. For example, the San Diego County town of Alpine, which has a population of about 13,000, is the only location that violates the eight-hour ozone standard. The county's other 2.8 million people—99.6 percent of the population—breathe air that meets both of EPA's ozone standards.

A detailed geographic analysis would be necessary for a precise estimate, but it is likely that EPA has overestimated by about a factor of two the number of people exposed to ozone in excess of the eight-hour standard. . . . The agency has confused a system for classifying non-attainment areas based on convenient political boundaries with a measure of actual air pollution exposure. Although EPA's trends report does highlight declines in emissions and pollution levels, it nevertheless greatly exaggerates the number of Americans exposed to polluted air.

The American Lung Association and PIRG also exaggerate the geographic extent of high air pollution levels through misleading countywide, or even statewide, summaries of air pollution data. Indeed, most areas given an "F" grade for air quality by the American Lung Association actually comply with EPA's one-hour ozone standard, and many comply with the more stringent eight-hour standard.

Bucking the trends

Air pollution, as noted earlier, has been on the decline for decades, and emission trends from vehicles and industrial sources confirm that pollution levels will continue to decline in the future. Yet activists have gone to great lengths to convince the public otherwise. One technique is to ignore long-term trends and instead highlight years in which air pollution levels rose when compared with the previous year.

For example, in "Danger in the Air," PIRG reported a 23 percent increase in eight-hour ozone exceedances between 2001 and 2002, while a recent National Environment Trust press release proclaimed "new survey finds massive smog problem in 2002." Ozone levels did indeed rise between 2001 and 2002, mainly because mild weather in 2001 made it an unusually low-smog year. In fact, despite a substantial overall decline in smog between 1990 and 2002, there were actually five years during this period in which ozone levels rose compared to the previous year in most parts of the country. Ozone levels are strongly affected by weather, which varies from year to year much more than pollution emissions. As a result, single-year changes in either direction cannot be used to infer long-term trends in air pollution. The national-average number of eight-hour ozone exceedances actually declined almost 50 percent between 1999 and 2000 because the weather in 1999 was unusually favorable to smog formation. This single-year change is as meaningless for inferring long-term trends as the rise in ozone between 2001 and 2002 highlighted by PIRG. Nevertheless, it is worth noting that large single-year decreases in air pollution have failed to inspire laudatory reports or press releases from environmental groups on the nation's success in fighting pollution. . . .

Figures show [that] among areas with the worst ozone, most achieved substantial pollution reductions during the 1990s, as did many areas with more modest pollution problems. The American Lung Association, PIRG, and other environmental groups simply omit air pollution trend data from their reports. . . . Regardless of annual fluctuations in smog levels caused by weather, the long-term trend is downward because pollution emissions from all sources continue to decline.

The future is clear

Although often unacknowledged by environmentalists, America's past success in combating air pollution actually occurred in spite of rapid growth in vehicle travel. For example, the substantial pollution reductions achieved since 1980 occurred at the same time that total vehicle-miles increased 75 percent. But can improvements in vehicle pollution control keep pace with increased vehicle use?

Environmentalists seem to think that pollution from vehicles will inevitably increase. They cite rising population, increased vehicle travel, and the popularity of sport-utility vehicles (SUVs), and conclude that air pollution will therefore increase in the future. For example, in "Clearing the Air with Transit Spending," the Sierra Club asserts that past pollution improvements are now being "canceled out" by SUVs and suburban development. Environmentalists appear to be unaware that technological progress is reducing automobile emissions far more rapidly than driving is increasing.

On-road pollution measurements show that average emissions from gasoline vehicles are declining by about 10 percent per year, even as SUVs make up an increasing fraction of cars on the road. Because of technological advances, newer cars continue to start out and stay cleaner as they age, when compared with previous models. EPA regulations that take effect with the 2004 model year require additional reductions of 70 percent for hydrocarbons and 80 percent for NOx below current new car standards, along with increased durability requirements. Similar regulations for diesel trucks require a 90 percent reduction in NOx and soot emissions starting in 2007, in addition to tougher NOx standards already implemented this year.

Although EPA's trends report does highlight declines in emissions and pollution levels, it . . . greatly exaggerates the number of American exposed to polluted air.

As far as SUVs are concerned, data from vehicle inspection programs and on-road emission measurements show SUV emissions have been converging with those of cars since the late 1990s. EPA's 2004 standards also make no distinction between SUVs and compacts; Chevy Suburbans must meet the same low emissions requirements as Geo Metros. Going forward, the growing popularity of SUVs will therefore make no difference for future air quality.

Based on observed emission trends and the requirements of new regulations, per-mile emissions will decline about 90 percent during the next 20 years, as twenty-first century vehicles make up an ever-larger portion of the fleet. Thus, even if Americans drive, say, 50 percent more miles 20 years from now (a greater increase than most metro areas project), total emissions would still decline by 85 percent from current levels.

Despite the evidence of substantial ongoing emission reductions from all major pollution sources, the American Lung Association asserts in its "State of the Air: 2003" report that "much air pollution cleanup has been stalled during the past five years" because of a lack of effort by EPA.

The dose makes the poison

Both the number of people affected by air pollution and the severity of the effects decline with decreasing exposure. Exposure depends not only on ambient pollution levels, but also on time spent outdoors and level of physical activity.

Epidemiologic studies have found permanent reductions in lung function in people exposed to several dozen days per year or more of ozone in excess of the one-hour standard. Environmentalists use those studies to claim that ozone remains a threat to lung development and long-term health. However . . . even in the most polluted areas, the number of high-ozone days each year is now only a fraction of past levels, suggesting that past studies are not applicable to current pollution levels. Indeed . . . hardly any areas of the country have ever had the frequent high ozone levels associated with irreversible reductions in lung function.

Short-term exposure to high ozone levels can also harm health. Studies with human volunteers have shown that ozone levels of about 120 ppb and above, especially when combined with exercise, can cause both decreases in objective measures of lung function and increases in subjective symptoms such as coughing and pain while breathing deeply. However, at moderate ozone levels—80 to 100 ppb—people generally do not experience measurable reductions in lung function or subjective respiratory symptoms. Laboratory studies have only found measurable respiratory effects at those ozone levels when subjects are exercising and exposed for more than two to three hours, even in people with pre-existing respiratory disease. Even here, many people are unaffected and the effects that do occur are transient and reversible, and do not harm long-term health. . . .

Environmental activists exaggerate the frequency and geographic extent of harmful pollution levels and also blur the distinction in health risk between modest and severe pollution problems. That misleads Americans to expect serious and permanent harm from current, relatively low levels of air pollution. For example, in "State of the Air," the American Lung Association asserts that 40 percent of Americans are "at risk" from ozone and suffer serious health damage even when ozone barely exceeds the eight-hour, 85 ppb benchmark just a few times per year, in spite of health research suggesting that this is a vast exaggeration.

Emission trends from vehicles and industrial sources confirm that pollution levels will continue to decline in the future.

PIRG's "Danger in the Air" declares without qualification that "our cities, suburbs and even our national parks are shrouded in smog for much of the summer," while the American Lung Association decries "the smog that regularly blankets many urban areas during the summer months," implying that most people are frequently exposed to air pollution at levels that could cause permanent harm. In reality, among areas exceeding federal ozone standards, the average location exceeds the one-hour benchmark about four times a year and the eight-hour benchmark about 11 times a year. Most areas of the United States now meet federal ozone standards, and high ozone levels have become infrequent in most areas that do exceed the standards. . . .

Getting real on air pollution

Activists and regulators do not produce reports and press releases on air quality for their own sake, but to influence public opinion. The reports . . . described above were accompanied by substantial public relations efforts, and often received coverage in many newspapers across the country. In most of those articles, reporters did not compare regulators' and activists' claims to actual pollution data and did not provide information on past trends and future prospects that would put the claims in context. As a result, activists and regulators have likely contributed to Americans' misperceptions on the state of the nation's air.

On-road pollution measurements show that average emissions from gasoline vehicles are declining by about 10 percent per year.

The battle against air pollution is actually a great success story in environmental protection and public health. The worst air pollution problems have been greatly reduced or eliminated, while parts of the greater San Bernardino and Fresno-Bakersfield areas in California are the only places that still frequently exceed the new eight-hour ozone benchmark. Rather than air pollution being a worsening national crisis, the vast majority of the country has attained the original federal health standards, and only a few regions are still a substantial distance from meeting the tougher new standards. Recent trends in ozone and particulate levels and in pollutant emissions, along with already-adopted new requirements, show that air pollution will continue to decline.

Whom the public trusts

Most Americans trust information from environmentalists and government agencies. A 1999 poll commissioned by the American Lung Association found that 90 percent of people trust environmental information provided by the association (59 percent of them a "great deal") while 79 percent trust EPA. A 2002 poll commissioned by the Sierra Club found that 57 percent of Americans trust environmental groups for information on environmental issues. As we have seen, that trust is misplaced.

Exaggerating health risks from air pollution can be as bad as minimizing them. Either extreme results in wasted resources and diversion of people's attention from more serious risks. Unwarranted alarmism also causes unnecessary public fear. The public's interest is in an accurate portrayal of risk. People ultimately bear regulatory costs through reductions in their disposable income because regulations increase the costs of producing useful goods and services. A large body of research shows that, on average, people use their disposable income to increase health and safety for themselves and their loved ones. A regulation will improve people's health only if the health benefits of the regulation exceed the harm caused by the regulation's income-reducing costs.

Regulators and environmentalists no doubt appear to be more credible sources of objective information when compared with, say, politicians or industry lobbyists. But, like other interest groups, the goals of regulators and activists often do not coincide with the interests of the vast majority of Americans. Environmental groups want to increase support for ever-more-stringent regulations and bring in the donations that support their activism. And while regulators want to show the success of their efforts to reduce air pollution, they also want to justify the need to preserve or expand their powers and budgets. Maintaining a climate of crisis and pessimism meets those institutional goals, but at the expense of encouraging the public to exaggerate its risk.

Air pollution levels, trends, and health effects are complex issues, yet journalists and editors face many constraints in trying to interpret environmental information for the public. Reporters often do not have specific subject expertise, and may not feel comfortable trying to sort out the nuances and complexities that lie behind proponents' portrayals of environmental data. Time and space limitations often prevent or discourage efforts to seek out experts who could critically evaluate particular claims.

Yet if the media are unable or unwilling to improve environmental reporting, the public is likely to remain misinformed. At the very least, reporters and editors must begin to treat claims by ostensible "do-gooders"—environmentalists, regulators, and even university researchers—with the same skepticism appropriate for other interested parties in regulatory debates.

5

Global Warming Caused by Air Pollution Will Harm Human Health

Jonathan A. Patz and R. Sari Kovats

Jonathan A. Patz is director of the Programme on Health Effects of Global Environmental Change at the Johns Hopkins Bloomberg School of Public Health in Baltimore, Maryland. R. Sari Kovats is codirector of the Centre on Global Change and Health at the London School of Hygiene and Tropical Medicine.

Air pollution, produced primarily by wealthy, energy-consuming nations, is using worldwide climate change. Global warming is now occurring at a faster rate than in any period over the past thousand years, and will have a serious impact on human health. Problems relating to climate change include heat waves and air pollution, a serious threat to health in cities; rising sea level, which will displace large populations in low coastal areas; river flooding, which will increase the spread of many diseases; drought and malnutrition, expected to increase; El Niño effects, which may cause weather extremes and the spread of disease; and highland malaria, expected to increase in some areas. Regions that already suffer environmental or socioeconomic stress are likely to face the greatest health threat; however, all countries will be affected.

Is climate change a serious threat to health? According to the most recent international assessments it unquestionably is, although its impact depends on where you live, your age, access to health care, and your public health infrastructure. Arguably, climate change is one of the largest environmental and health equity challenges of our times; wealthy energy consuming nations are most responsible for the emissions that cause global warming, yet poor countries are most at risk. In a globalised world, however, the health of populations in rich countries is affected as a result of international travel, trade, and human migration. Mapping "hotspots" of ecological risk has proved to be a useful construct for prioritising and focusing resources to stem the threat of losing biodiversity. Similarly, identifying hotspots in climate change and human health may help public health practitioners in anticipating and preventing any additional burden of disease. . . .

Recent and projected climate change

According to the United Nations Intergovernmental Panel on Climate Change, evidence of recent warming is building. Since the late 1950s, the global average surface temperature has increased by 0.6°C, snow cover and ice extent have diminished; during the past century, the sea level has risen on average by 10–20 cm and the temperature of the oceans has increased. Mid-range estimates for future climate change are 3°C global mean warming and a rise in the sea level of 45 cm by 2100. Increased variability in the hydrological cycle (more floods and droughts) is expected to accompany global warming. The rate of change in climate is faster now than in any other period in the past thousand years.

Although climate warming and changes in precipitation are expected to affect higher latitudes disproportionately, hotspots in health and climate change will occur where human populations are already at risk from climate extremes (such as drought induced famine or flooding) and lack adequate health infrastructure. Such vulnerable hotspots may therefore not necessarily coincide with areas that are experiencing the greatest change in climate. For any given vulnerable region, adverse health effects will generally occur in poor populations that have little capacity to adapt, predominantly in the tropics and subtropics.

Impacts of climate change will occur in the context of other environmental and socioeconomic pressures. For example, heavy precipitation can more readily cause dangerous flooding in areas denuded of forests. Localised warming can be intensified in sprawling cities through the "urban heat island" effect. The impact of increases in extreme rainfalls will be exacerbated by impervious road surfaces and inadequate drainage, making cities more prone to flooding. Impacts on food resources will compound current overharvesting of fisheries and intensive animal production.

Hotspots of climate change and health

The strategy of mapping hotspots has been used by conservationists to choose locations to which to apply limited resources so that the world's biodiversity is best preserved. Impacts do, however, occur at the local level, and identifying vulnerable regions or countries does not account for diverse regional texture.

Hotspot 1—Heat Waves or Air Pollution

This kind of hotspot consists of geographically expanding or sprawling cities, replacing vegetation with surfaces retaining heat. Also cities with poor quality housing that currently experience an urban heat island effect, and cities that have topography that gives rise to stagnant air masses and summer pollution are at risk (for example, Santiago [Chile] and Mexico City [Mexico]).

Mortality generally increases at both high and low temperatures above and below an optimum temperature value. Populations in warmer regions tend to be sensitive to low temperatures, and populations in colder climates are sensitive to heat. Vulnerability to heatwaves is driven by socioeconomic factors such as poor housing. Cities in developing countries may therefore be more vulnerable to heatwaves, although little research has been done in these countries. Elderly people and people with pre-existing illnesses are disproportionately affected. Mortality is primarily due to cardiovascular, cerebrovascular, and respiratory disease. A heatwave in Chicago in 1995 caused 514 heat related deaths (12 per 100 000 population). The urban heat island effect, whereby urban areas experience higher and nocturnally sustained temperatures owing to the concentration of heat retaining surfaces (for example, asphalt and tar roofs), can amplify general warming trends.

Increased ambient temperature and altered patterns of wind and air mass can affect chemistry in the atmosphere. Temperature and the formation of ozone at ground level (photochemical urban smog) are related: a strong positive relation with temperatures above 32°C has been observed in some US cities. Ozone can heighten the sensitivity of people with asthma to allergens and contribute to the development of asthma in children. The impact of climate change on the future frequency of episodes of air pollution during the summer in a given city remain highly uncertain.

Wealthy energy consuming nations are most responsible for the emissions that cause global warming, yet poor countries are most at risk.

Hotspot 2—Sea Level Rise
This type of hotspot consists of settlements on low lying deltas or coral atolls and coastal megacities (such as Cairo, Egypt). After a rise in sea level, widespread flooding, intrusion of salt water, and coastal erosion are expected in low lying coastal settlements. The number of people at risk from flooding by coastal storm surges is projected to increase from the current 75 million to 200 million in a scenario of mid-range climate changes, in which a rise in the sea level of 40 cm is envisaged by the 2080s. Countries such as Vietnam, Egypt, Bangladesh, and small island nations would be especially vulnerable.

Coastal communities may experience forced migration of populations. Thirteen of the world's 20 current megacities are situated at sea level. Rising seas could result in salination of coastal freshwater aquifers and disrupt stormwater drainage and sewage disposal. [Researchers R.] Nicholls and [S] Leatherman showed that the extreme case of a rise of one metre in the sea level could inundate low lying areas, affecting 18.6 million people in China, 13 million in Bangladesh, 3.5 million in Egypt, and 3.3 million in Indonesia. Considering the health burden experienced by refugees and populations subjected to overcrowding, lack of shelter, and competition for resources, the problems presented by displaced populations may turn out to be the largest public health challenge regarding the global health effects of climate change. Conflict may be one of the worst results emerging from such forced migration.

Hotspot 3—Flooding
This type of hotspot consists of regions prone to river flooding, such as Central America, Europe, South Asia, and China. Specific watersheds in many countries throughout the world would be affected. Climate change may increase the risk of flooding of rivers. Immediate effects are largely death from drowning and injuries caused by being swept against hard objects. Medium term effects include increases in communicable diseases caused by ingestion of contaminated water (for example, cholera or hepatitis A) and contact with flood waters (for example, leptospirosis). Outbreaks of leptospirosis . . . occurred after floods in Nicaragua and Brazil. In Bangladesh in 1988, watery diarrhoea in a population displaced by floods was the most common cause of death for all age groups under 45, followed by respiratory infection. In Bangladesh, settlement of populations in high risk areas such as floodplains and river deltas increases vulnerability.

Heavy rainfall and runoff influences the transport of other microbial and toxic agents from agricultural fields, human septic systems, and toxic dumps. Rainfall can alter the transport and dissemination of microbial pathogens (such as cryptosporidia and giardia), and temperature may affect their survival and growth.

Hotspot 4—Drought and Malnutrition
This kind of hotspot consists of areas currently experiencing food insecurity and risk of drought, together with a lack of resources to import food (for example southern and eastern Africa, parts of Latin America, and central Asia). The UN Intergovernmental Panel on Climate Change projects a reduction in crop yields in most tropical and subtropical regions caused by mid-continental droughts. Some crops in tropical locations would be decimated because many are already grown in climate conditions near their maximum temperature tolerance. Africa and parts of Latin America are considered to be the most vulnerable regions.

The rate of change in climate is faster now than in any other period in the past thousand years.

Decreased availability of water as a result of climate change could affect populations in the subtropics where water is already scarce. [In 2002] about a third of the world's population (1.7 billion people) live in water stressed countries, and that number is projected to increase to 5 billion people by 2025. Decreases in annual average streamflow are anticipated in central Asia and southern Africa, and the food supply may be affected. Politically inflexible regimes can exacerbate climate crises, as may have occurred during the . . . severe drought in North Korea [in 2003].

Despite technological advances such as improved crop varieties and irrigation systems, agricultural productivity depends largely on weather conditions. According to the UN Food and Agriculture Organization (FAO), 790 million people in developing countries are malnourished. Nearly half the populations of countries in central, southern, and eastern Africa are already undernourished, and these regions are highly vulnerable. In addition, diarrhoea and diseases such as scabies, conjunctivitis, and trachoma are associated with poor hygiene and result from a breakdown in sanitation if water resources become depleted.

Hotspot 5—El Niño Effects

This hotspot consists of regions that experience weather extremes associated with the El Niño weather pattern[1] (for example, Peru and Ecuador for floods; southern Africa, Indonesia, and Malaysia for drought; and some areas for epidemics of infectious disease, such as malaria in Punjab or cholera in Bangladesh). Some evidence shows that stronger or more frequent El Niño events may accompany global warming.

Climate change is likely to lead to greater extremes of drying and heavy rainfall and increases the risk of droughts and floods that occur with El Niño in many regions. Studies have shown that the El Niño cycle in certain areas is associated with changes in the risk of diseases transmitted by mosquitoes, such as malaria and dengue fever, and diseases caused by arboviruses, other than dengue virus. The risk of malaria in areas in South America, Central Asia, and Africa has been shown to be sensitive to variability in climate driven by El Niño. In Peru, more children develop diarrhoeal disease when temperatures are high, and admissions during the El Niño of 1997–8 increased appreciably. In Southeast Asia, episodes of hazardous air pollution from fires in Indonesia were related to drought conditions connected with El Niño.

Hotspot 6—Highland Malaria

This kind of hotspot consists of areas situated at the fringe of regions where malaria is endemic (for example, East Africa). Vectorborne disease such as malaria and dengue fever, are generally more influenced by ambient conditions than are diseases passed directly from human to human. Arthropods—such as mosquitoes, ticks, and fleas—are cold blooded and therefore sensitive to subtle changes in temperature and humidity. Populations of non-human mammalian hosts, such as rodents, are affected by conditions of their habitat and the weather. . . .

Many of the highland regions in Africa that are surrounded by lowland areas where malaria is endemic are densely populated. Small changes in the distribution of malaria may therefore expose large numbers of people to infection. Some malaria epidemics in the African highlands have been associated with abnormally warm or wet weather conditions. The areas of the highlands of Africa that are currently free of malaria therefore represent an ecological zone of special concern, where the distribution of malaria may potentially be affected by climate warming.

The way forward

Medical practitioners can consider these hotspots of climate change and health as a guidepost for understanding populations and people at most risk from climate change. Doctors' awareness of current health needs in their region is the key to identifying potential health problems that can be exacerbated by more extreme climate variability and long term climate change. Disease monitoring in such hotspots is a priority in order to prevent further health problems.

---

1. "El Niño" refers to an unusually warm ocean current that sometimes occurs along the western coast of South America. It prevents upwelling of nutrient-rich cold, deep water, and disrupts regional and global weather patterns.

Many options for limiting greenhouse gas emissions are available in the short and medium term. Policy makers can encourage energy efficiency and other climate friendly trends in the supply and consumption of energy. Key consumers of energy include industries, homes, offices, vehicles, and farms. Efficiency can be improved in large part by providing an appropriate economic and regulatory framework for consumers and investors. . . .

Efficiency and equity

The United States contains 5% of the total population of the world yet produces 25% of total annual emissions of greenhouse gas. This discrepancy exemplifies the ethical implications posed by climate change. A country's ability to cope with the impacts of climate change depends on its wealth, technology, and general infrastructure. Impoverished populations in the developing world do not have the industry, transportation, or intensive agriculture that cause global warming, yet they have limited capacity to protect themselves against the adverse consequences. In this way, climate change is one of the largest challenges of our times for environmental and health equity. If developing nations do not choose development pathways using more efficient energy technology, the imbalance of "equity" may be lessened—but the global warming problem will be exacerbated greatly.

6

Global Warming Caused by Air Pollution Will Not Harm Human Health

Thomas Gale Moore

Thomas Gale Moore is a senior fellow at the Hoover Institution, an organization dedicated to limiting government intrusion into the lives of individuals.

There is no evidence that future climate change, caused by the emission of greenhouse gases, will be harmful to human health. Claims that tropical and insect-spread diseases, heat-related deaths, and violent storms will dramatically increase are unfounded. According to the World Health Organization, health levels have improved dramatically worldwide and will continue to improve in the future. The historical record shows that the human population is actually healthier during warm periods of time, so rather than adversely affecting human health, global warming is likely to be beneficial.

In promoting the Kyoto Protocol[1], which would require a major cut in greenhouse gas emissions, the White House claims that "scientists agree that global warming and resulting climate disruptions could seriously harm human health (projections include 50 million more cases of malaria per year)". [Former] President [Bill] Clinton has asserted: "Disruptive weather events are increasing. Disease-bearing insects are moving to areas that used to be too cold for them. Average temperatures are rising. Glacial formations are receding."

In his 1997 exhortation to the environmental ministers at Kyoto, [former] Vice President Al Gore warned that "disease and pests [are, will be?] spreading to new areas." The White House's home page continues that

---

1. In 1997 more than 150 nations, including the United States, negotiated this treaty aimed at reducing worldwide carbon dioxide emissions. In 2001 the United States withdrew its support for the treaty.

Thomas Gale Moore, *In Sickness or in Health: The Kyoto Protocol Versus Global Warming.* Stanford, CA: Hoover Institute, 2000. Copyright © 2000 by the Board of Trustees of the Leland Stanford Junior University. Reproduced by permission.

theme: Americans better watch out; global warming will make them sick.

The Sierra Club has also weighed in, asserting that "doctors and scientists around the world are becoming increasingly alarmed over global warming's impact on human health. Abnormal and extreme weather, which scientists have long predicted would be an early effect of global warming, have claimed hundreds of lives across the US in recent years. Our warming climate is also creating the ideal conditions for the spread of infectious disease, putting millions of people at risk."

The Public Interest Research Group, a left-leaning environmental organization, fears "Health Threats—Climate change is projected to have wide-spread impacts on human health resulting in significant loss of life. The projected impacts range from increased incidence of illness and death due to heat stress and deteriorating air quality, to the rise in transmission rates of deadly infectious diseases such as malaria, dengue fever, and hanta virus." Other environmentalists and health experts have also forecast that global warming would bring death and disease.

Little cause for alarm

Not only does my own research demonstrate that the claims of imminent doom are unwarranted, but other studies have founded little cause for alarm. Knowledgeable organizations, such as the World Health Organization and the American Medical Association have ignored the subject, suggesting that, in their eyes, it is unimportant.

After examining the potential impact of global warming on poor countries, the American Council on Science and Health (ACSH) took a realistic view and reported that

> Nearly all of the potential adverse health effects of projected climate change are significant, real-life problems that have long persisted under stable climatic conditions. Bolstering efforts to eliminate or alleviate such problems would both decrease the current incidence of premature death and facilitate dealing with the health risks of any climate change that might occur.

> Policies that weaken economies tend to weaken public health programs. Thus, it is likely that implementation of such policies would (a) increase the risk of premature death and (b) exacerbate any adverse health effects of future climate change.

As the ACHS concludes:

> From the standpoint of public health, stringently limiting such emissions [greenhouse gases] at present would not be prudent. Fossil-fuel combustion, the main source of human induced greenhouse-gas emissions, is vital to high-yield agriculture and other practices that are fundamental to the well-being of the human population. A significant short-term decline in such actions could have adverse health repercussions.

The optimal approach to dealing with [the] prospect of climate change would (a) include improvement of health infrastructures (especially in developing countries) and (b) exclude any measures that would impair economies and limit public health resources.

The World Health Organization's *World Health Report 1998: Life in the 21st Century*, gave the globe an A for progress. The WHO showed that remarkable advances have been made in increasing life spans, decreasing disease and suffering, and improving health for virtually all age groups and that the future looks even rosier. To quote the Executive Summary: "As the new millennium approaches, the global population has never had a healthier outlook."

How can this be? After all, the White House tells us the next century promises to be one of rising temperatures, spreading disease, and increasing mortality. Somehow, the WHO didn't get the word. The *World Health Report 1999: Making a Difference* again fails to address this problem that the White House believes is so worrisome.

According to the [World Health Organization], the only significant and growing threat to human health is HIV/AIDS, a disease that has nothing to do with climate.

According to the WHO, the only significant and growing threat to human health is HIV/AIDS, a disease that has nothing to do with climate. Indeed, we have made substantial progress in controlling many major infectious diseases. By 1980, for example, smallpox had been eradicated; yaws had virtually disappeared (except to medical students, even the name of this tropical skin disease is unfamiliar). As a result of antibiotics and insecticides, the threat of plague has declined; improvements in sanitation and hygiene have made outbreaks of relapsing fever rare. Unbelievably, for those who remember summers of fear and polio insurance, poliomyelitis is scheduled for eradication. . . .

A look to the future

Looking to the future, the WHO report identifies three global trends affecting health—none is global warming. One is economic: the WHO reports (1998) on the "unparalleled prosperity" between 1950 and 1973, which resulted in marked improvements in health and life expectancies. The organization identifies the years since 1993 as another era of economic "recovery," which has once again contributed to reduced mortality. The other trends singled out as having significant health effects are population growth and social developments, particularly urbanization.

Over the last forty years, the growth in the world's economy has brought about a doubling of the world's food supply, while the number of human mouths has grown much more slowly. This has led to a decline in the proportion of people who are undernourished. Since 1970, literacy rates have increased by more than 50 percent. Physical well-being has also grown apace. More people have access to clean water, sanitation facilities, and minimum health care than ever before. Like the 1999 review, prior World Health Reports largely ignored global warming as a significant threat to the health and well-being of the globe's population. And rightly so.

Of the 50 million plus deaths in 1997, about one-third stemmed from infectious and parasitic diseases, most of which have nothing to do with climate. The remaining deaths were from such killers as cancer, circulatory diseases, and prenatal conditions, none of which would be aggravated by a warmer world. Most infectious and parasitic diseases are unrelated to climate.

The WHO has identified AIDS, one of the most devastating afflictions, as a growing menace in Africa, but it bears no relationship to temperature or rainfall. Only insect-spread diseases, such as malaria and dengue fever, and diseases like cholera and typhoid that are spread through contaminated water, could be worsened by climate change (and then only if swampy polluted areas were allowed to expand without thought to sanitation, window screens, and other precautions that have all but eradicated those diseases in the northern latitudes).

But bear these statistics in mind: In the developed world, as recently as 1985, infectious and parasitic diseases accounted for 5 percent of all deaths; in 1997, they caused only 1 percent of all deaths. In short, even for such insect-borne diseases as malaria, climate is much less important than affluence. Singapore, located two degrees from the equator, is free of that dreadful malady, while the mosquito-carried scourge is endemic in rural areas of Malaysia, only a few hundred miles away. Singapore's healthy state stems from good sanitary practices that reduce exposure. The wealth of the island-state allows it to maintain an effective public health program.

The frightful forecasts of an upsurge in disease and early mortality stemming from climate change are unfounded, exaggerated, or misleading.

Nor should we be overly concerned with the diseases spread by mosquitoes in tropical areas. If climate change were to occur, according to the global warming models, the poles would warm more than the equator while temperatures would increase more in the winter and at night than during the day. In consequence, the tropics, including Africa, would warm less than the United States or Europe. Any increased burden on health in Africa or southern Asia would, therefore, be small.

With or without climate change, public sanitation should be emphasized as the most effective means of attacking water- and insect-borne diseases everywhere. A warmer world will not add significantly to morbidity in Third World countries. A poorer world most certainly will.

Both the scientific community and the medical establishment assert that the frightful forecasts of an upsurge in disease and early mortality stemming from climate change are unfounded, exaggerated, or misleading and do not require reducing greenhouse gas emissions. *Science* magazine reported [in 1997] that "predictions that global warming will spark epidemics have little basis, say infectious-disease specialists, who argue that public health measures will inevitably outweigh effects of climate". The article added: "Many of the researchers behind the dire predictions concede that the scenarios are speculative."

Global warming as currently forecast by the International Panel on Climate Change (IPCC) would not bring tropical diseases to Americans or shorten their lives or inflict more violent storms bringing death and destruction to the United States. Moreover, the warmer climate predicted for the next century is unlikely to induce a rise in heat-related deaths. As the article in *Science* magazine points out, "people adapt. . . . One doesn't see large numbers of cases of heat stroke in New Orleans or Phoenix, even though they are much warmer than Chicago."

Tropical diseases

Concern about tropical and insect-spread diseases is overblown. Inhabitants of Singapore, which lies almost on the equator, and of Hong Kong and Hawaii, which are also in the tropics, enjoy life spans as long as or longer than those of people living in Western Europe, Japan, and North America. Both Singapore and Hong Kong are free of malaria, but that mosquito-spread disease ravages nearby regions. Modern sanitation in advanced countries prevents the spread of many scourges found in hot climates. Such low-tech and relatively cheap devices as window screens can slow the spread of insect vectors. The World Health Organization notes:

> until recent times, endemic malaria was widespread in Europe and parts of North America and . . . yellow fever occasionally caused epidemics in Portugal, Spain and the USA. Stringent control measures . . . and certain changes in lifestyle following economic progress, have led to the eradication of malaria and yellow fever in these areas.

Under the stimulus of a warmer climate, insect-spread diseases might or might not increase. Many of the hosts or the insects themselves flourish within a relatively small temperature or climatic range. Plague, for example, spreads when the temperature is between 66° and 79° with relatively high humidity but decreases during periods of high rainfall. Higher temperatures and more rainfall are conducive to an increase in encephalitis. Malaria-bearing mosquitoes flourish under humid conditions with temperatures above 61° and below 95°. Relative humidity below 25 percent causes either death or dormancy.

Parasitic diseases, such as AIDS, Lyme disease, yellow fever, malaria, and cholera, can usually be controlled through technology, good sanitary practices, and education of the public. Even without warming, it is certainly possible that dengue fever or malaria could invade North America. Unfortunately, some of the government's well-meaning environmental policies may make the vector more likely. The preservation of wetlands, although useful in conserving species diversity, also provides prime breeding grounds for mosquitoes that can carry these diseases. If the United States does in the future suffer from such insect-borne scourges, the infestation may have less to do with global warming than with the restoration of swampy areas. . . .

Deaths in winter versus summer

Recent summers have sizzled. Newspapers have reported the tragic deaths of the poor and the aged on days when the mercury reached torrid levels. Prophets of doom forecast that rising temperatures in the next century portend a future of calamitous mortality. Scenes of men, women, and children collapsing on hot streets haunt our imaginations.

Heat stress does increase mortality, but it affects typically only the old and the infirm, whose lives may be shortened by a few days or perhaps a week. There is no evidence, however, that mortality rates rise significantly. The numbers of heat stress–related deaths are very small; in the United States; the number of deaths due to weather-related cold exceeds them. During a recent ten-year period, which includes the very hot summer of 1988, the average number of weather-connected heat deaths was 132, compared with 385 who died from cold. Even during 1988, more than double the number of Americans died from the cold rather than from the heat of summer. A somewhat warmer climate would clearly reduce more deaths in the winter than it would add in the summer.

A somewhat warmer climate would clearly reduce more deaths in the winter than it would add in the summer.

Humans also seem to be able to adapt to hot weather. Adjusting for demographic differences and economic factors, people in cities with hot climates enjoy longer life spans than those in cold areas. A warm climate does not increase mortality. Moreover, the spread of air-conditioning reduces the discomfort of extremely high temperatures. . . .

Hurricanes and tornadoes

Typically, global-warming prophets claim that climate change will increase the threat from more frequent or violent storms. Their argument, which has some plausibility, is that a warmer climate means that more heat energy will be trapped in the atmosphere, leading to bigger and stronger weather systems. On the other hand, warming is most likely to be greatest near the poles and less at the equator. The strength of weather systems is actually a factor of the differential in temperatures between the two regions. Since this differential will diminish, so too will the likelihood of more intense cyclones.

Major weather disasters do kill. The evidence, however, simply fails to support the proposition that weather is becoming more violent. In the Atlantic basin, the number of intense hurricanes, those scaled between three to five (five being the most violent), has actually declined during the 1970s and 1980s. The four years from 1991 to 1994 enjoyed the fewest hurricanes of any four years over the last half century. Researchers have found that the average number of tropical storms and hurricanes has not changed over the previous 52 years, while there has been a major *decrease* in the number of intense hurricanes.

For the Pacific around Australia, other researchers have found that the number of tropical cyclones has *decreased* sharply since 1969/70. Of the ten deadliest hurricanes to strike the continental United States, all raged prior to 1960, notwithstanding the huge expansion of population in coastal areas vulnerable to such storms. . . .

History shows benefits of warm weather

History demonstrates that warmer is healthier. Since the end of the last Ice Age, the earth has enjoyed two periods that were warmer than the twentieth century. Archaeological evidence shows that people lived longer, enjoyed better nutrition, and multiplied more rapidly in warm periods than during epochs of cold. . . .

Although it is impossible to measure the gains exactly, a moderately warmer climate would likely benefit Americans in many ways, especially in health. Contrary to many dire forecasts, however, the temperature increase predicted by the IPCC [Intergovernmental Panel on Climate Change] under a doubling of greenhouse gases, which is now less than 4.5°F, would yield health benefits for inhabitants of the United States.

In summary, If the IPCC is correct about a warmer climate over the next hundred years, Americans and probably Europeans, the Japanese, and other people living in high latitudes should enjoy improved health and extended lives. High death rates in the tropics appear to be more a function of poverty than of climate. Thus global warming is likely to prove positive for human health.

7

Indoor Air Pollution Is a Major Risk to Public Health

John Manuel

John Manuel is a freelance writer based in Durham, North Carolina, specializing in energy and environmental health topics.

Indoor air pollution is a serious health hazard in the United States. Carbon dioxide, the most dangerous indoor air pollutant, comes primarily from improperly used heating appliances, particularly unvented heaters. Studies have also shown adverse health effects from a number of volatile organic compounds, including formaldehyde, chlorination by-products, and polybrominated diphenyl ethers, that are frequently found at unhealthy levels in many buildings. Additional indoor health threats come from mites and molds, and from indoor dust, found to some extent in every home. Many older homes also contain lead and asbestos, which are hidden but serious hazards. While indoor air pollutants cannot be completely eliminated, there are a variety of measures that can be taken to detect and reduce them, including ventilating, eliminating moisture, and cleaning house regularly.

Over the past seven years, the Science Advisory Board of the U.S. Environmental Protection Agency (EPA) has consistently ranked indoor air pollution among the top five risks to public health. This is a sobering thought, given that people in the United States spend an average of 90% of their time indoors and that many intrinsically associate home with safety and comfort. Although stories about hazards such as lead paint and asbestos in older, deteriorating homes have become commonplace, people may be surprised to learn that environmental problems can plague even the most modern homes. "Environmental health hazards occur in houses of all ages," says John Bower, cofounder of The Healthy House Institute, an independent resource center for designers, architects, contractors, and homeowners, and an editorial advisory board member for the *Indoor Environment Review*. "They just tend to be of a different nature."

Building science specialists cite a number of trends that make the in-

John Manuel, "A Healthy Home Environment?" *Environmental Health Perspectives*, vol. 107, July 1999.

door environment, particularly indoor air quality, a growing concern. Since the energy crisis of the 1970s, builders have concentrated on building tighter homes as a way of minimizing heating and air-conditioning costs. Tighter houses can be healthy houses, but more care must be taken to avoid generating or trapping pollutants indoors, where they can accumulate to hazardous levels.

Another energy-conscious trend is the growing popularity of ventless gas heaters. The trend started with freestanding kerosene heaters, which were purchased for millions of households during the energy crisis, and now includes ventless natural gas space heaters, fireplaces, and gas logs. Aside from the combustion gases they produce, these devices release one gallon of moisture for every 100,000 British thermal units (BTUs) of energy[1] they consume each hour. Excess moisture in a home is a haven for the growth of molds and fungi, which may cause a variety of allergic, infectious, and toxic reactions in humans.

Modern building materials, furnishings, and paint and other coatings can . . . be a source of indoor air pollution.

Modern building materials, furnishings, and paint and other coatings can also be a source of indoor air pollution. Often these materials are made with volatile organic compounds (VOCs) that outgas into the home, sometimes causing respiratory problems. Wall-to-wall carpeting can serve as a reservoir for pollutants, including pesticides, tracked in from outdoors, as well as for dust mites, bacteria, and asthma-inducing allergens. Even household water may not be completely safe—radon gas, a cause of lung cancer, can become aerosolized in water droplets in hot showers, and water may contain chlorinated by-products associated with elevated rates of bladder cancer and adverse reproductive outcomes.

The carbon connection

There are dozens of potential environmental health hazards in the home but the most dangerous are combustion gases. Oil- and gas-fired furnaces, water heaters, ovens, wood stoves, charcoal grills, and fireplaces all produce combustion gases. These gases may include carbon monoxide (CO), carbon dioxide, nitrogen dioxide, nitric oxide, sulfur dioxide, water vapor, hydrogen cyanide, formaldehyde, and various hydrocarbons.

By far the most hazardous of these is CO. In 1997, the American Association of Poison Control Centers' Toxic Exposure Surveillance System reported 20,930 cases of CO poisoning from all known sources, including 191 life-threatening cases and 37 fatalities. CO is formed when a carbon-containing fuel such as kerosene, charcoal, wood, or gasoline, is incompletely burned. Natural gas in the United States does not contain carbon, but CO may form if the gas is burned without an adequate air supply.

CO is colorless, odorless, and tasteless, which makes its presence all

---

1. a standard measurement for energy

but undetectable to humans without the use of special equipment. When breathed, CO combines with hemoglobin to form carboxyhemoglobin (COHb), which disrupts the flow of oxygen to the body and brain. CO's potential to kill is well known, but the bigger story may be how many people suffer adverse health effects from chronic and often undetected exposure to low levels of the gas. Symptoms of CO poisoning, which include fatigue, headache, dizziness, nausea, and vomiting, so closely mimic the common cold that exposures may not be properly diagnosed. . . .

Symptoms of CO poisoning . . . so closely mimic the common cold that exposures may not be properly diagnosed.

In addition to causing flu-like symptoms, studies show that chronic exposure to low-level CO may also cause poor vision, retinal hemorrhaging, and behavioral impairment. . . .

Anecdotal evidence and a number of studies point to faulty or improperly used heating appliances as the primary source of CO in the home. A study of unintentional CO poisoning by Magdalena Cook and colleagues at the Colorado Department of Health, published in the July 1995 issue of the *American Journal of Public Health*, traced 478 of 981 poisonings to faulty furnaces (363 cases), kerosene or space heaters (27 cases), gas appliances (72 cases), and fireplaces (16 cases). (The other cases were related to inhalation of smoke from fire and auto exhaust.) Common causes of furnace-related CO exposure include cracked heat exchangers, backdrafting of the furnace flue caused by depressurization, or blockage of the chimney. The study did not determine whether the kerosene or other space heaters or gas appliances were faulty or not. The report did state, "With the onset of colder weather, malfunctioning furnaces may be turned on, and kerosene or space heaters may be inappropriately used in enclosed spaces."

The problem with kerosene space heaters is that they are unvented; thus, they dump all their combustion by-products into the living space. A study by Ron Williams, a former senior research associate with Environmental Health Research and Testing in Research Triangle Park, North Carolina, published in the September/October 1992 issue of *Indoor Environment* (the former journal of the International Association for Indoor Air Quality), found that the use of unvented kerosene heaters in mobile homes caused a significant rise in indoor CO concentrations, sometimes in excess of the U.S. air exposure standard of 9 parts per million (ppm) CO over an eight-hour period.

Unvented heaters

Health officials are also concerned about the rising popularity of unvented natural gas appliances intended for use as supplemental heaters. According to the Vent-Free Gas Products Alliance, 1,250,000 ventless gas appliances were sold in the United States in 1998. Citing research performed by the American Gas Association research division, the alliance claims that properly sized and installed vent-free products used for no more than four continuous hours conform to "reasonable" indoor air quality guidelines set by various government agencies for CO, nitric oxide, carbon dioxide, and water vapor. However, critics say it is unreasonable to assume that all or even most of these appliances will be properly sized, used only for supplemental heating, and provided with sufficient makeup air. In a recent study by the Manufactured Housing Research Alliance, 7 of 12 manufactured homes using ventless kerosene heaters and 4 of 7 homes using liquid propane heaters were out of compliance with American National Standards Institute emission rate standards for CO. The study, titled *Manufactured Housing Fuel Switching Field Test Study*, also found that in five homes the owners operated their vented gas fireplace logs with the damper closed in order to "get more heat" out of the gas logs.

Thomas Greiner, an extension engineer with Iowa State University in Ames, has performed hundreds of indoor air quality investigations in the United States and abroad. "I've been into too many homes that use these unvented heaters as the primary source of heat," Greiner says. "I also find that as you get into colder climates, people use a larger-sized heater than is called for in the specifications. There's also a question as to whether the occupants are letting in enough outside air to dilute the combustion by-products. My opinion is that these heaters are a real step backwards [from] the goal of improved air quality in the U.S."

Anecdotal evidence and a number of studies point to faulty or improperly used heating appliances as the primary source of CO in the home.

Michael Calderera, associate director of technical services for the Gas Appliance Manufacturers Association, based in Arlington, Virginia, counters that a distinction should be made between an unvented kerosene heater and an unvented natural gas space heater. An unvented natural gas space heater employs a device called an oxygen detection safety (ODS) pilot system, which monitors the level of oxygen in the room and automatically shuts off the supply of gas to the unit if the level of oxygen drops below a level set by the national product safety standard. ODS devices became a requirement of the national product safety standard in 1980. Since that time, says Calderera, "Over seven million unvented space heaters have been installed in the United States and, as far as we know, there has not been a single documented death resulting from emissions from an ODS-equipped unit."

Problems can occur in homes when gas ovens are used as supplemental or primary heating sources. Examining a survey of customers of the Con Edison utility company in New York City who have natural gas stoves but not natural gas heating systems, researchers observed that more than half of the 340,000 customers were using more gas than was deemed normal for cooking use. The researchers subsequently visited 120 of these homes and found that in 50% of them the occupants were using the gas range as a supplemental source of heating. Only 12% of these stoves had hoods with working exhaust fans that could eliminate stove-produced pollutants, and only 3% had working window fans. In an article published in the February 1981 issue of the *Journal of the Air Pollution Control Association*, author T. D. Sterling and colleagues concluded that a large number of urban dwellers may be chronically exposed to gas range-produced indoor pollutants, which may, in turn, result in ill health effects.

Volatile visitors

Dozens of different VOCs have been measured in indoor air from a variety of sources including building products, cleaning agents, paints and finishes, fragrances and hair sprays, office equipment such as copiers and printers, and infiltration of outdoor air. Concentrations of VOCs measured indoors are usually far below occupational threshold limit values (TLVs), the point above which health effects may occur, but they may at times, exceed human odor thresholds, or the point at which an odor becomes offensive. A few compounds, principally aldehydes, are suspected of causing adverse health effects, but because many VOCs haven't been studied, no one knows what their effects might be.

One VOC that has been studied extensively and that is a cause of great concern in the home is formaldehyde. Formaldehyde-based resins are widely used in building materials (subflooring and paneling), furniture, and cabinets. Consumer products such as permanent-press fabric, wallpaper, and fingernail polish and hardeners can also emit formaldehyde. "By far the worst nonwood-product emissions came from acid-cured floor finishes," says Thomas J. Kelly, a senior research scientist at Battelle in Columbus, Ohio, who compared emission rates of formaldehyde from materials and consumer products in California homes in an article published in the 1 January 1999 issue of *Environmental Science and Technology*. "Even after 24 hours of drying," wrote Kelly, "each coat emitted at a steady state that as 5–10 times higher than emissions from the very worst wood product."

Airborne formaldehyde can act as an irritant to the conjunctiva and upper and lower respiratory tract. Symptoms of short-term exposure are temporary and, depending upon the intensity and length of exposure, may range from burning or tingling sensations in the eyes, nose, and throat to chest tightening and wheezing. Acute severe reactions may be associated with hypersensitivity, a condition of hyperreactive airways that effects 10–20% of the U.S. population, according to the EPA. . . .

Another type of VOC, chlorination by-products, can result when public water supplies are treated with chlorine. Some of these by-products are suspected carcinogens. Public health officials have calculated risk assessments based primarily upon exposure through ingestion of cold water. However, recent studies claim that humans are exposed to these chemicals through various means that include bathing and showering, and that the risks may have been underestimated. In a study published in the January 1996 issue of *EHP*, Clifford Weisel, an associate professor at the Environmental and Occupational Health Sciences Institute at Robert Wood Johnson Medical School in Piscataway, New Jersey, and colleagues determined that people are exposed to chloroform and trichloroethene through inhalation and dermal absorption [through the skin] as well as ingestion during daily bathing and showering. Weisel's studies showed that exposure through showering is roughly equal to that from drinking water. However, as to how much the former route of exposure contributes to adverse health effects, Weisel says, "At the moment, we don't understand the biological mechanisms of action well enough to establish risk estimates. The delivered dose of the metabolite varies by route of exposure, and that can affect the potential outcome." Weisel's article calls upon public health officials to raise their risk assessments to include these routes of exposure.

Biological pollutants are found to some degree in every home, school, and workplace.

Concern has been expressed . . . about a possible threat to human health from exposure to polybrominated diphenyl ethers (PBDEs) in the home. PBDEs are . . . compounds that can accumulate in human tissue. Their metabolites have been shown to interfere with the thyroid system. PBDEs are used as flame retardants in high-impact polystyrene, flexible polyurethane foam, textile coatings, wire and cable insulation, and electrical connectors. In consumer products, PBDEs are typically used in interior parts and incorporated into the polymer matrix, which minimizes the potential of exposure to the public. However, new evidence raises concerns that PBDE vapors might emanate from television sets and be absorbed by human tissue.

In a paper published in volume 35 of *Organohalogen Compounds* and presented at "The 18th Symposium on Halogenated Environmental Organic Pollutants," held in Stockholm in August 1998, Jacob de Boer, director of the DLO-Netherlands Institute for Fisheries Research, and colleagues examined the case of a male Israeli citizen who suffered from headaches, painful lesions, dizziness, and other symptoms after prolonged television watching in a small, unventilated room. Blood samples taken after the onset of these symptoms revealed chromosomal abnormalities consistent with chemical exposure. Ten years after the exposure, sampling of both the subject's adipose tissue [connective tissue where fat is stored] and the television set revealed the presence of PBDEs. While proof of a relationship could not be established, the authors hypothesize that exposure to vapors from the television set may have played a role in the observed health effects.

"I think PBDEs are the sleeper compounds of the future," says Larry Robertson, a professor of toxicology at the University of Kentucky in Lexington and a coauthor of the article. "They are slowly but irrevocably accumulating in human tissue." Robertson says more research is needed to determine how these compounds break down in the environment.

Of mites and molds

Biological pollutants are found to some degree in every home, school, and workplace. They come from outdoor air in the form of pollen and other allergens, from human occupants who expel viruses and bacteria, from pets that shed dander, from insect pests, and from moist surfaces that allow mold and fungi to grow.

In the publication *Indoor Air Pollution—An Introduction for Health Professionals*, the EPA cites a number of factors that allow biological agents to grow and be released into the air. High relative humidity (more than 50%) encourages dust mite populations to increase and allows fungal growth on damp surfaces. Damp carpeting as well as moisture from inadequate ventilation of bathrooms and kitchens can promote mite and fungus contamination. Appliances such as humidifiers, dehumidifiers, air conditioners, and drip pans under cooling coils can also support the growth of bacteria and fungi. Finally, components of heating, ventilating, and airconditioning (HVAC) systems may serve as reservoirs of microbial growth and distribution. The EPA states in its online publication *Biological Pollutants in Your Home* that 30–50% of all structures in the United States and Canada have damp conditions that may permit the growth and buildup of biological pollutants.

Biological agents in indoor air are known to cause infections, hypersensitivity, and toxic effects. The EPA indicates that allergic reactions may be the most common health problem with indoor air quality in homes. Such reactions can range from mildly uncomfortable to life-threatening. Allergic reactions to dust mites are particularly problematic. Bower's book *The Healthy House* states that dust mite allergy affects approximately 10% of the U.S. population. Several studies have shown that exposure to house dust mite allergens is associated with asthma in susceptible children. . . .

Dirty dusting

The expression "dusting the house" may conjure an image of a housewife with a feather duster, whisking the lampshades and tables to give them an extra shine. But studies in recent years indicate that house dust is often not so benign and that the health problems it can cause are nothing to sniff at.

House dust contains all manner of particles from such activities as cooking, other household processes, and smoking. It may also contain pollutants brought in from outdoors such as pollen, pesticides, and heavy metals, some of which are known or suspected human carcinogens. Outdoor pollutants are tracked in on shoes or brought in on clothing or the fur of household pets. In fact, concentrations of pesticides and other outdoor organic pollutants may be higher inside the house than outside.

"We've found concentrations of pesticides . . . 10–100 times higher in carpet dust than in yard soils," says Robert G. Lewis, a senior scientist with the National Exposure Research Laboratory of the EPA in Research Triangle Park. "And these compounds last far longer indoors than they do out of doors. In a study we did in 1990, we found DDT [an insecticide that is toxic to animals and humans] to be the highest in concentration of all particles found in the dust of an old carpet. DDT use was banned in the United States in 1972."

Lewis says young children who spend lots of time at floor level are at the greatest risk for exposure to such chemicals by ingestion and inhalation of resuspended house dust, which exists at highest concentrations close to the floor. "We don't have risk criteria on many of these compounds in dust and we don't know what the bioavailability is once the dust is ingested or inhaled," Lewis says. "But given that most pesticides are toxic to humans and some are potentially carcinogenic, we should try to limit our exposures by whatever means."

Hidden hazards

Radon. Radon, a colorless, odorless gas found to varying degrees in soil and subsurface water, is a pollutant that has received a great deal of attention in recent years. The EPA estimates that radon pollution is responsible for up to 20,000 lung cancer deaths each year. The agency has prepared a map of the United States showing the geologic potential for radon in different parts of the country; however, no region of the nation should be considered entirely safe. Most of the time, radon gas leaves the soil and dissipates into the atmosphere, but it can be drawn into the living space of a house through leaky floors or duct systems. As radon starts to decay, it gives off a series of radioactive particles that can damage lung tissue if inhaled. Radon is measured in units of picocuries per liter. The EPA suggests that people exposed to more than 4 picocuries per liter in the home should take remedial action to remove the source of radon.

Lead and asbestos. Two other materials, lead and asbestos, may be a problem in older homes. Lead was commonly used in household paints up to the 1950s, when its use began to decline. In 1978, the CPSC banned the manufacture of house paint containing more than a trace amount (0.06%) of lead. Lead is highly toxic and has been linked to a variety of neurodevelopmental problems among children living in older homes with peeling or chipping lead paint. Exposure comes through children either eating the chips directly or crawling on carpets contaminated with lead dust and then putting their hands in their mouths. According to Bower, when children eat paint chips, the majority of the lead is excreted because the chips are fairly large. However, when children eat dust, the majority of the lead is absorbed, making lead dust a more dangerous hazard.

Asbestos is a mineral that was commonly used for insulating hot water pipes in homes built between 1920 and 1972. It was also used as a component in joint finishing and patching compounds, in the backing of vinyl, asphalt, and rubber flooring, and in textured ceilings. If inhaled, asbestos fibers can lodge in the lungs and lead to a variety of diseases including lung cancer and asbestosis, a chronic fibrotic lung disease. Recognizing its dangers, manufacturers eliminated asbestos from most building products by the 1970s, and its use in household products was banned by the CPSC in 1977. Still, older homes may have asbestos in some locations and it can become hazardous if the materials begin to deteriorate and become airborne.

Cleaning house

People who have the luxury of building their own home can now employ a wide variety of measures and materials to minimize their potential exposure to indoor environmental hazards. Such materials range from ventilation tubes that purge radon gas from the crawl space, to electrical heating and hot water systems that do not emit combustion gases, to steel kitchen cabinets that do not emit VOCs. However, the vast majority of people in the United States live in homes that are not custom-built to avoid such environmental health problems. A number of strategies can help people avoid adverse health effects within the home. For homes that have gas- or oil-fired heating systems, experts recommend yearly servicing by a qualified heating technician. Gas stoves and ranges should only be operated with the exhaust fan turned on. If the range lacks an exhaust system, one should be installed. Many building science experts recommend against using ventless gas-fired heating systems in the home. If these are used, experts recommend they be operated in accordance with manufacturer instructions and for only a few hours at a time. Experts also recommend that CO detectors be installed in every home.

The EPA recommends that every homeowner and every condominium owner living below the third floor have his or her home tested for radon, either by a professional or using a radon kit (available in most hardware stores). Long-term (90-day) testing kits are recommended, as radon concentrations can fluctuate at different times of the year. If high levels of radon are found in the home, several strategies can be pursued including ventilating the living space, sealing off the floor from the crawl space or basement, and depressurizing the subfloor through the use of vents and fans.

Concentrations of pesticides and other outdoor organic pollutants may be higher inside the house than outside.

For people sensitive to VOCs, the EPA recommends limiting the use of personal items such as scents and hair sprays; household products such as rug and oven cleaners; paints, lacquers, and finishes; dry-cleaning fluids; office equipment such as copiers and printers; office products such as correction fluids and graphics materials; and craft materials such as glues and adhesives. If new carpeting, paints, or finishes containing formaldehyde are installed or applied, the home should be well ventilated for several days afterward. Pesticides and biocides that emit VOCs should only be used outdoors and should be stored outside the living space.

Experts say the best strategy for avoiding the buildup of mold and mildew is to reduce moisture levels in the home. Exhaust fans should be used in bathrooms and kitchens, where high levels of moisture are produced. Clothes dryers should be vented outside the house. Roof or plumbing leaks should be repaired immediately. Humidifiers and drip pans for HVAC [heating, ventilation, and air conditioning] systems should be cleaned regularly. Flood-damaged carpets, draperies, or furniture should be thrown out.

Dust mites require food, water, and moderate temperatures for growth. The EPA advises maintaining a low relative humidity (below 45%) in the home, vacuuming often and, if necessary, using EPA-approved pesticides. Mattresses are a prime haven for dust mites because they are made of fluffy materials and they are a site of extended human exposure (dust mites feed off of skin flakes). Allergists recommend that both mattresses and box springs be covered with special covers made of tightly woven material or plastic. Bedding should be washed in water of at least 130°F.

Airborne pollutants cannot be totally eliminated from the home, but they can be kept to a minimum. Health officials warn against smoking indoors. Air filters in HVAC systems should be changed monthly. If occupants continue to suffer allergic reactions to pollens and other allergens, experts say a more sophisticated filtration system may need to be installed. High-efficiency particulate accumulator (HEPA) filters remove 99% of particles larger than 0.3 microns, which includes pollens and household dust. . . .

While vacuuming is always recommended to reduce the biologicals, pesticides, and heavy metals that can build up in carpets, studies show that standard housecleaning strategies are often not sufficient to significantly reduce these pollutants. In order to improve indoor air quality, cleaning must be thorough and well thought out. Deborah Franke, a senior research scientist with Research Triangle Institute, an independent research laboratory in Research Triangle Park, and colleagues analyzed the effectiveness of routine and improved housecleaning methods against dust, bacteria, fungi, and VOCs in an institutional building in North Carolina. Their findings, published in the December 1997 issue of *Indoor Air*, include a list of procedures most effective in improving indoor air quality. These include the use of HEPA vacuum cleaners with high-efficiency bags and filters, hot-water extraction cleaning methods in the deep cleaning of carpets, the use of disposable damp cloths for dusting and mopping, low VOC-emitting cleaning agents, and interior doormats to trap and collect particles at entrances.

Unlike outdoor air quality, which is protected by the Clean Air Act and other legislation, the responsibility for clean indoor air falls primarily on the individual. Although information on hazardous indoor air exposures is often lacking (for example, manufacturers may not be required to list all of the chemicals that are contained in household products), the homeowner is not without resources. Information is available on the World Wide Web and through many publications produced by the EPA, the CPSC, and private organizations such as The Healthy House Institute. Given the amount of time spent indoors, ensuring a healthy home environment may soon become a quest for everyone—not just homeowners—to consider.

8

Air Pollution Is a Serious Health Risk in Asia

Charles W. Petit

Charles W. Petit is a contributing writer for U.S. News & World Report.

A huge cloud of air pollution stretches across much of India, Bangladesh, and Southeast Asia, threatening the health of billions of people living in that region. The thick layer of dust, ash, and smoke from fires and industry causes a large number of respiratory illnesses each year. Scientific evidence also shows that the pollution may be causing drought and famine. Researchers are beginning to realize that Asia's pollution, because it spreads for thousands of miles, is a global health threat.

V. "Ram" Ramanathan sat on an airliner heading south from Bombay. Ahead were the Maldives, an archipelago near the equator, where the atmospheric scientist from the Scripps Institution of Oceanography near San Diego planned to set up instruments to study haze and weather. He expected that results from the international project would come slowly and be of interest only to specialists. He was not prepared for what he saw just gazing out the plane window.

As he took off from Bombay, the layers of brown gunk in the sky were no surprise. Pollution controls on factories and vehicles are rare in his native land. Hundreds of millions of its citizens burn low-quality coal, wood, and cow dung for cooking and heating. But nearly 1,000 miles later over the open sea, the dirty pall still had not given way to blue sky and white clouds. "The haze just kept going and going. It didn't even seem to thin out. I was thinking, this is something big."

It is. Since Ramanathan's 1998 flight, scientists have realized that the pall he saw is just part of a vast brown cloud that often extends thousands of miles east, across China. A stew of dust, ash, and smoke from fires and industry, the cloud threatens the health of the billions who live under it. The fine particles, or aerosols, also warm some areas and cool others, drying up storm clouds and perhaps even shifting India's life-giving monsoon. In many places the haze swamps greenhouse gases as a climate-changing force, say scientists. The atmospheric havoc in Asia may even play a role in El Niño, the climate cycle now [in 2003] drenching the southern United States.

Brown cloud over Asia

Much of this picture is still fuzzy, but scientists are working to sharpen it. Ramanathan and his Scripps colleague Paul Crutzen, a chemist and Nobel laureate, made a start with their Indian Ocean Experiment in the late 1990s, which studied haze from a score of ground stations and from aircraft. Their glimpses of the cloud's extent and impacts helped set off an explosion of similar studies across India, off Japan and Korea, and in China, which has launched the largest single scientific project in the country's history to analyze aerosols and climate. And it has spawned a new United Nations effort called Project Asian Brown Cloud. Led by Ramanathan and Crutzen, it is organizing a massive study of the pollution's sources and effects, and what to do about it.

In a way, Asia with its dirty, fast-growing industry is repeating on a far vaster scale the smoky evolution of European and U.S. industry in the 19th and early 20th centuries. Coal consumption in China, for example, was 50 percent higher than in the United States in 1999 and could be twice as high by 2010. Across Asia, coal heats houses and cooks meals. Smoke from agricultural burning and wildfires adds to the brew. In China, the haze sometimes starts as dust blowing off western deserts, "but it picks up all kinds of toxic pollutants as it travels," says F. Sherwood Rowland, a University of California–Irvine chemist who received a Nobel Prize for work on ozone. "We can detect Asian aerosols blowing all the way across the U.S."

A stew of dust, ash, and smoke from fires and industry, the cloud threatens the health of the billions who live under it.

Yet just five years ago, Ramanathan could be startled by the pall he saw from the plane window because experts still thought of smog outbreaks as local, covering a city or filling a river valley. Until recently nobody had seen the goop all in one glance. Cameras on early weather satellites were calibrated for clouds but not hazes. But new full-color satellite camera systems now send images of a nearly continuous, 2-mile-thick blanket of sulfates, soot, organic compounds, dust, fly ash, and other crud draped across much of India, Bangladesh, and Southeast Asia, including the industrial heart of China.

The sand-colored air of Los Angeles is pristine by comparison. When Chinese scientists told U.S. colleagues about foul air back home, "we'd say we have smog here too," says Lorraine Remer, who analyzes satellite data at NASA's Goddard Space Flight Center. "Then we saw the extinction numbers"—satellite data on how much the brown cloud dims light. Across much of Asia, they were several times higher than anything ever seen in American smog. "We were standing there not believing it," she says. In and around India, the researchers found sunlight was reduced by 10 percent. Crop scientists say this is enough to reduce rice yields by 3 percent to 10 percent across much of the country. Ground data in China show the same thing. In Beijing, airborne particulates are routinely five times as high as in Los Angeles. Donald Blake, an atmospheric chemist at the University of California-Irvine, says that a colleague on a visit asked a group of kindergartners to draw the sky. They all reached for the gray crayon.

It's worse than unsightly. India has 23 cities of more than 1 million people; not one meets World Health Organization pollution standards. Indoor smoke from poorly vented fires is blamed for half a million premature deaths annually in India alone, mostly women and children. In southern China and Southeast Asia, as many as 1.4 million people die annually from pollution-related respiratory ills.

Disturbing effect

Researchers are coming to realize that, through a long chain of effects, the brown cloud may also be to blame for drought and flooding. Scientists' understanding of how aerosols shape climate is not nearly as well developed as it is for greenhouse gases like carbon dioxide, still No. 1 on any list of human impacts on climate. "But one common aspect," says Ramanathan, "is that the haze and its heating of the atmosphere is sufficient to disturb climate a lot."

Unlike the whiteish sulfate particles from cleaner-burning power plants in the United States and Europe, the Asian hazes are dark with soot. As a result, they absorb sunlight and can double the rate at which it warms the atmosphere several thousand feet up, while shading and cooling the ground below. Some scientists think that the net effect is to boost global warming. But the more certain impact of the hazes is on rainfall, says Jeff Kiehl of the National Center for Atmospheric Research in Boulder, Colo. "They are radically changing the temperature profile of the atmosphere in many areas, with a big impact on where rain falls and how much."

India has 23 cities of more than 1 million people; not one meets World Health Organization pollution standards.

By cooling the northern Indian Ocean, the haze reduces evaporation, cutting the water supply for rainfall. On land, the warm air aloft acts as a lid on cloud formation, quashing the convection that feeds thunderstorms. And the aerosols themselves seed the formation of tiny mist particles—so many that they suck water out of the air and choke off the growth of larger drops that would fall as rain. While the haze particles dry out the land, the rain does fall over the sea, where larger, natural sea-salt particles promote droplet growth. "We're shifting rain from the land to the ocean," says Daniel Rosenfeld of the Hebrew University of Jerusalem.

At least that's the theory, and there are signs it may be happening. Some computer climate models predict that the hazes over India should displace the annual monsoon rains, leading to floods in the south and east of the country while drying the north and shrinking the vital Himalayan snowpack. "That's just the pattern we are starting to see emerge," says Surabi Menon of the Goddard Institute for Space Studies in New York City.

Changing weather patterns

In southeastern China, where haze has cut sunlight by 2 percent to 3 percent every 10 years since the 1950s, temperatures are dropping, while rising elsewhere in the country, presumably because of greenhouse gases. The changed temperature patterns have rerouted storm tracks, one recent Chinese study said. The study blamed the shift for severe floods in the nation's south in recent years, coupled with drought in the north. It ranked the new weather pattern as the greatest sustained change in China's climate in more than 1,000 years. Some scientists also suspect that the pollution cloud could be cooling the sea surface and slowing evaporation in the far western Pacific, off Asia. The effects could ripple across half the globe to the United States, because the western Pacific is the breeding ground for El Niños, the bouts of Pacific warming that change rainfall across the Americas and beyond.

All of this is enough to make Asia's brown cloud, and the sparser hazes elsewhere, into a global climate threat. Fortunately, hazes are far easier to counter than greenhouse gases like carbon dioxide. Clean up industry and smother the fires, and in a few weeks rain would wash the skies clean. Carbon dioxide, in contrast, lingers for centuries, and ordinary pollution controls can't touch it.

Some scientists, distressed at the reluctance of the U.S. government and many developing nations to tackle greenhouse gases, hope that the relatively easier task of curbing fine particles could kickstart international efforts to address climate change. Going after hazes, particularly those heavy with soot, is "a no-lose situation as far as I'm concerned," says Stanford University atmospheric researcher Mark Jacobson.

The Chinese government, rattled by the data on the country's polluted air, is doing just that. For both health and weather reasons, it has largely replaced home use of coal with cleaner-burning natural gas in big cities and is starting to require catalytic converters on vehicles. China also hopes to restore blue skies to Beijing in time for the 2008 Olympics.

9

Pollution Regulation Reforms Will Worsen Air Quality

John Edwards

John Edwards, elected to the U.S. Senate in 1998, serves on the Committee on Health, Education, Labor, and Pensions; the Committee on Small Business; and the Select Committee on Intelligence.

Changes to the New Source Review provisions of the Clean Air Act will increase air pollution in the United States. Poor air quality is already a serious problem affecting the health of Americans. These changes will alter the way pollution levels are calculated, allowing increased air pollution by industries. Before any changes are implemented, additional studies should he conducted to assess their potential effect. Protecting human health through clean air should be a top priority for the administration.

Editor's Note: The Clean Air Act's New Source Review provisions regulate the construction and maintenance of major emitting industrial facilities. In 2003 the Environmental Protection Agency made several controversial changes to these rules, which will allow modifications of some existing sources of air pollution without subjecting them to new emission standards.

For months the Administration has talked about massive changes in clean air protections and for months senators on both sides of the aisle have said to the Administration: Before you go through with these changes, would you please tell us in detail how these changes are going to affect our families? In other words, would you please look before you leap?

We have been asking that question for months, and for months the Administration has refused to answer. On November 22 [2003], they went ahead with their massive changes without telling us how it was going to affect the health of the American people.

I believe the Administration does not want to share these facts because they are afraid of what the facts will show. They are afraid people will see what their rule changes will do. When you study these rules, when you lis-

John Edwards, address before the U.S. Senate, Washington, DC, January 21, 2003.

ten to the experts, you will see that they will make our air dirtier. These rules will add more soot to our cities and more smog to our national parks. At the end of the day, these rules will allow more kids to get asthma attacks, more seniors to have heart problems which land them in the emergency room, and more people will lose their lives prematurely.

This amendment[1] is a very modest response to these proposed changes. It does not block the rules forever. It does not put them off for years. It just says, let's put these rules off for about six months and use that time to determine how these changes will affect human health, how they will affect kids with asthma, senior citizens with cardiorespiratory problems. It seems to be a perfectly reasonable thing to do. I hope my colleagues will support the amendment.

These [new] rules will allow more kids to get asthma attacks, more seniors to have heart problems which land them in the emergency room, and more people will lose their lives prematurely.

We are saying, let's get a study from the nonpartisan, completely respected National Academy of Sciences. That is all we are talking about—a six-month delay to look at these changes to see, before they go into effect, what effect they will have on the health of the American people.

The science of pollution is completely clear. Pollution causes heart and lung problems. It aggravates asthma. It causes the smog that ruins the view in our Nation's parks. It causes premature deaths.

According to Abt Associates, a nonpartisan research group, just 51 powerplants are responsible for more than 5,500 deaths every year, for over 106,000 asthma attacks, and for costs to our economy of between $31 billion and $49 billion. That is only 51 powerplants. If you did the same study of other industries, the numbers would go up dramatically.

North Carolina has some of the worst pollution in the country. According to Dr. Clay Ballantine, a physician in Asheville in western North Carolina, just living and breathing in western North Carolina costs one to three years off the average life of a person. The University of North Carolina School of Public Health found that in many of our counties three in 10 kids have asthma, which is three times the national average.

Just walking in the Great Smoky Mountains is as bad for your lungs as breathing in many big cities. When the head of the EPA [Environmental Protection Agency], Christie Todd Whitman, visited the Great Smokies last Fourth of July [2002], she could barely see 15 miles at a place where you used to be able to see 75 to 100 miles. So clean air is a huge priority. It is important for our kids, for seniors, and for our parks.

This Administration has made radical changes in the regulations under the Clean Air Act. This is about a program called New Source Review

---

1. This amendment would have placed a six-month delay on implementation of changes to the New Source Review, a program that regulates the construction and maintenance of major emitting industrial facilities. The amendment was defeated and changes to the New Source Review were implemented in 2003.

or NSR. The basic idea of NSR is simple. Under the Clean Air Act, if some-one builds a new factory, the new factory has to have state-of-the-art equipment to prevent pollution, but there is a special deal for factories that were built before 1977. Those factories don't need to install new pollution controls unless and until their toxic emissions go up by a significant amount. Only when that happens does the plant have to install these new controls that others have to meet instantly. This is what the New Source Review is all about.

There is no question—all of us believe—reforming NSR is a good idea. We ought to do two things: One, we ought to cut red tape, which is a problem; two, we ought to cut pollution.

Under Carol Browner, EPA Administrator in the Clinton Administration, positive work was done in that direction. But the debate today is not about those kinds of reasonable and sensible reforms that are in the best interest of the American people. This debate is about this Administration's package.

There are several glaring problems with that package. First, the Administration developed these rules through a series of secret consultations with executives from power and oil companies. It would not have been so bad if the Administration had also been talking secretly to regular patients and kids and doctors about what effect these changes in the rules would have on their lives and their health. But there is no evidence they did that. Instead, the Administration focused on one side and favored that side in the changes they made in the rules.

Premature deaths and asthma attacks cost our country over $30 billion each year. The costs of cleaning the air are a small fraction of that amount.

The second problem is this Administration has never explained in any serious way whether these changes will in fact harm human health, whether they will cause more pollution, more asthma, or more premature deaths. For months we have asked for a serious qualitative study, and for months we have not received that study. . . .

On November 22, 2002, the Administration just went ahead, finalized the rules without giving any credible evidence on what impact this would have on human health.

Let me give two examples of what these rules will do:

First, the rules change the way pollution levels are calculated. Under the New Source Review, a factory has to clean up only if it increases its pollution level. It matters a lot how we measure the factory's initial pollution level, what's called the "baseline." Up to now, the rule has been that the baseline is the average for the last two years—that is the basis on which we determine whether there has been an increase in pollution, unless the company can prove another period is more representative of recent emissions. But the basic rule has been that you establish the baseline by looking at the last two years. That makes sense.

What this Administration proposes doing makes no sense. What they are saying is, instead of using the last two years we let the factory choose any two years out of the last 10. So instead of looking at the last two years as a baseline to determine whether emissions have gone up, what they are saying is we are going to let the factory choose any two years in the previous 10 in order to determine whether emissions have gone up.

So even if the reality is that their pollution level is quite low right now, they get to go back a decade and say that pollution is high.

They can even take emissions from accidents and malfunctions and use those to inflate their baseline. And because they can make pollution 10 years ago look like pollution today, they can pollute even more without cleaning up.

You don't have to take my word for it. According to internal documents, career staff at the EPA said that this change would "significantly diminish the scope" of the New Source Review. A study by the Environmental Integrity Project found that at just two facilities, the new rules would allow over 120 tons of the pollution into the air. The National Association of State and Local Air Regulators says that this change "provides yet another opportunity for new emissions to avoid NSR." So the bottom line is more pollution.

Here is a second example. The new rules contain something called a "clean unit" exemption. In theory, the exemption should give companies an incentive to clean up by giving them benefits if they install state-of-the-art technology. It is a perfectly good idea. But this Administration has provided an exemption as long as the company installed new equipment anytime during the last 10 years. In other words, if a company did something good in 1994, they get a free pass to increase pollution in 2003, nine years later.

Again, this makes no sense. Again, it will increase pollution. Again, here is what the State and local air commissioners said. This rule "would substantially weaken the environmental protections offered by the NSR program."

Now, when it comes to the effects of these rules, it is true that the State administrators could be wrong. The career officials at EPA could be wrong. I could be wrong. We could all be wrong. The rules could be okay.

But even if we are all wrong—and I do not believe we are—shouldn't we get the whole story and get a real answer to the question before putting our kids and our seniors at risk?

Six months is not a long time to wait in order to get the whole story. It is far better to wait six months than to say to this Administration, go ahead, roll the dice. It is okay. We are willing to put the lives of our children and seniors at risk, and we are willing to let this rule go into effect even though we do not know what effect it is going to have on the health of our seniors and children.

Opposition to reform

Let me talk for a minute about the broad opposition to these rules.

This Administration likes to talk about State flexibility, but these regulations take flexibility away from the States and force some States to lower their protections. Again, this is the view of the State experts: "The revised requirements go beyond even what industry requested. . . . Because the reforms are mandatory, they will impede, or even preclude, the ability of States and localities all across the country to protect the air. Although our associations believe NSR can be improved . . . [w]e firmly believe the controversial reforms EPA is putting in place . . . will result in unchecked emission increases that will degrade our air quality and endanger public health."

That is the States. Now listen to the doctors. Over a thousand doctors from all across the country have urged this Administration not to go ahead with these final rules. These doctors see the effects of air pollution every day in their practices and in the emergency rooms, and they warned that "it is irresponsible for the EPA to move forward in finalizing new regulations that could have a negative impact on human health."

This is not a partisan issue. The State air quality folks are not partisans. The local air quality folks are not partisans. And then there's Republicans for Environmental Protection, a group to which 12 past or present former Republican Members of Congress are connected. Republicans for Environmental Protection recently wrote a letter supporting my amendment.

They wrote that "a reasonable delay (of the rules) is necessary in order to allow independent researchers to investigate how the New Source Review revisions would affect emissions and the resulting impacts on public health." So Republicans support this amendment as well.

We will hear people say that protecting the air is too expensive. But at the 51 powerplants I mentioned earlier, premature deaths and asthma attacks cost our country over $30 billion each year. The costs of cleaning the air are a small fraction of that amount. So clean air not only saves lives; it also saves money. . . .

This amendment is about final rules. It is a very modest amendment. It will protect our kids from asthma, our seniors from heart problems, our parks from smog. This amendment will make sure we look before we leap. I urge my colleagues on both sides of the aisle to support this amendment.

10
Pollution Regulation Reforms Will Improve Air Quality

Christopher Bond

Christopher Bond, the governor of Missouri from 1972 to 1976 and from 1980 to 1984, was first elected to the U.S. Senate in 1986. He serves on a number of committees, including the Committee on Appropriations and the Committee on Environment and Public Works.

Changes to the New Source Review provisions of the Clean Air Act will reduce air pollution in the United States. The New Source Review has hindered industry and needs to be reformed. The changes will allow companies the flexibility they need to upgrade their facilities, and will cause reductions in ozone, smog, and other hazardous pollutants. In addition to environmental progress, economic performance and energy conservation will be improved.

Editor's Note: The Clean Air Act's New Source Review provisions regulate the construction and maintenance of major emitting industrial facilities. In 2003 the Environmental Protection Agency made several controversial changes to these rules, which will allow modifications of some existing sources of air pollution without subjecting them to new emission standards.

I believe the Administration's New Source Review reforms[1] are good for the environment, good for energy security, and good for the economy. I think it is important for my colleagues to understand that the EPA's [Environmental Protection Agency] New Source Review reforms will improve air quality and benefit the environment. EPA has already done the environmental analysis. It shows that four of the five provisions in the final rule will reduce air pollution. That is correct. I said "will reduce air pollu-

1. The New Source Review is a program that regulates the construction and maintenance of major emitting industrial facilities. The proposed reforms to the program were passed in 2003.

Christopher Bond, address before the U.S. Senate, Washington, DC, January 21, 2003.

75

tion." The other provision will have no significant effect on air quality. NSR will no longer stand as a barrier to facilities installing state-of-the-art pollution control technology. Anybody who has been around Washington very long knows the law of unintended consequences. We do things we think are going to help, and they turn out to be a hindrance.

The New Source Review, as it has worked, has been a hindrance because companies cannot make routine improvements and upgrades to their facilities to make them operate more efficiently, take less energy, burn less fuel, emit less pollution or polluting substances, anywhere from volatile organic compounds to the other emissions from powerplants. They do that because the New Source Review says that anytime you want to do anything significant on a major plant, you have to go through the whole process. It takes a very long time, and you are required to make very significant upgrades beyond what the available dollars in the company would sustain.

The NSR [New Source Review] reforms will . . . cut hazardous air pollutants and ozone-depleting substances. Our families will suffer fewer cases of premature mortality, asthma, and other respiratory diseases.

The incremental continuing improvements, day by day or actually month by month or even year by year, cannot be made because of NSR. If you change it the way the EPA administrator has proposed, NSR will no longer stand as a barrier to facilities installing state-of-the-art pollution control technology.

Pollution reduction

The NSR reforms that EPA has proposed will actually cut emissions of tens of thousands of tons per year of volatile organic compounds. NSR reforms will reduce ground-level ozone and smog. The NSR reforms will also cut hazardous air pollutants and ozone-depleting substances. Our families will suffer fewer cases of premature mortality, asthma, and other respiratory diseases.

I would say further that EPA's NSR reforms are good for the Nation's energy security. Why? Simply because they will allow facilities to install modern technologies which use energy more efficiently. We all ought to be able to agree on that. Using energy efficiently conserves energy, and reduces the polluting byproducts of energy production. The facilities will be able to reduce their energy consumption, reduce their dependence on foreign energy sources, and reduce our Nation's dependence on foreign energy supplies.

What is wrong with that? In our current troubled times, we should not stand in the way of any proposal which reduces our dependence on foreign and Middle Eastern oil. I would also say that the EPA NSR reforms are good for the economy. Companies would now be able to make rapid changes to meet their changing business climates without getting bogged down in time-consuming government red tape.

Company flexibility

The reforms will continue to protect the environment while giving companies the flexibility they need to get new products to the market quickly. We have all of the elements that should go into a forward-looking environmental program. We have made great progress, but we have also developed glitches in our system, and anybody who has thought about the system knows that we need to make it more efficient. We need to rationalize it. We need to give it flexibility so environmental improvements can be made with the least hassle.

I am talking about environmental improvements. That is what this NSR proposal does. It allows not only energy conservation, improved economic performance, but environmental progress as well. What is wrong with that?

I have yet to hear what is the objection to providing better environmental performance in a way that is flexible, that encourages companies to move forward. This is such a good idea that the last administration supported it. You heard me right. This was one of their proposals.

The reforms EPA finalized this winter were actually proposed in 1996 during the Clinton Administration by EPA Administrator Carol Browner. I thought it was a good idea then; I think it is a good idea now. The only change is there is a new administration, with a different President [George W. Bush].

I hope this is not the reason behind some of my colleagues seeking to raise the issue and challenge it. If it was a good idea in the Clinton Administration, does it become a bad idea in the Bush Administration? I don't think so.

I think we are on the right track with what the Clinton Administration started. The NSR reforms are good for the environment, they are good for energy security, and they are good for the economy.

11

A Global Approach to Pollution Regulation Is Necessary

Christopher G. Reuther

Christopher G. Reuther is a contributing writer for Environmental Health Perspectives.

Around the world there is a growing recognition that air pollution problems cannot be solved locally. Instead, because of the way pollution flows across international borders, many countries are acknowledging that prevention efforts need to be coordinated globally. There have been a number of international agreements on limiting transported air pollutants, and many other discussions and agreements on limiting transported air pollutants are taking place around the world, as international governments increasingly approach air pollution in a borderless context.

The acid rain in Lorraine comes partially from Spain. Similarly, about half the acid rain that falls on Canada originates in the United States, as does a large portion of the ground-level ozone found there. Air pollution never respects international boundaries, but in [2000] a spate of meetings and agreements has shown international governments to be more willing than ever to try to limit the amount of their air pollution that drifts into other countries. Recently, nations have begun working harder to identify who exports and who imports the air pollutants that flow across international borders—and who should bear the burden of cleaning the global atmosphere.

In February 2000, the United States and Canada began discussing how to expand their existing bilateral air pollution agreement to include ozone. At a March 20–25 meeting of the United Nations Environment Programme (UNEP) in Bonn, Germany, an agreement on persistent organic pollutants (POPs) was discussed. The goal is to sign a POPs convention in May 2001, which would effectively result in the first-ever global

Christopher G. Reuther, "Winds of Change," *Environmental Health Perspectives*, vol. 108, April 2000.

convention on transboundary air pollution.[1] Perhaps even more significant, last December [1999] the nations of the United Nations Economic
Commission for Europe (UNECE) signed a comprehensive agreement to
limit the export of pollutants that cause several environmental problems—acid rain, ground-level ozone, and the eutrophication of waters. . . .

Sulfur dioxide (SO_2), nitrogen oxides (NO_x), volatile organic compounds (VOCs), POPs, particulate matter, and heavy metals are all now being discussed in international forums. Unlike greenhouse gases and ozone-
depleting substance—for which global agreements exist—many of these
air pollutants were once thought to be problems that could be solved locally, where the effects occur. Behind this policy shift are increasing emissions in some parts of the world, better monitoring, and an improved understanding of air pollution transport. "There is a growing recognition that
for these air issues, any national government that attempts to deal with
the problem alone will meet with only limited success because they are the
kinds of problems that require collective action," says John Buccini, director of the Commercial Chemicals Evaluation Branch of Environment
Canada and chairman of the UNEP POPs convention negotiations.

---

*"There is a growing recognition that for these air
issues, any national government that attempts to
deal with the problem alone will meet with only
limited success."*

"The problems that we are facing are becoming less of a regional char-
acter . . . and more and more of a northern hemispheric or global charac-
ter," says Henning Wuester, a UNECE official and member of that group's
secretariat for its Convention on Long-Range Transboundary Air Pollution. "There is now science showing that pollution travels much further
than previously anticipated." Some models have suggested, for example,
that POPs released into the air in China will show up in Canada three to
five days later.

According to the World Health Organization (WHO), air pollution
causes 2.7 million deaths per year. While many of these are caused by indoor air pollution, the WHO estimates that just eliminating ground-level
ozone could save 180,000 lives annually (including 5,000 in the United
Sates) and reduce suffering for millions of people with asthma and other
respiratory ailments. Reductions in emissions of sulfur oxides and particulate matter could save 500,000 lives, according to the WHO. These common air pollutants can also cause defoliation of trees and acidification of
soil, as well as other detrimental ecosystem effects. The Ozone Transport
Assessment Group of the U.S. Environmental Protection Agency (EPA) estimates on their Frequently Asked Questions site that ground-level ozone
causes damage to U.S. crops totaling $2–3 billion each year.

---

1. The Stockholm Agreement on Persistent Organic Pollutants (POPs) was signed by 150 nations,
including the United States, in May 2001, and a number of these nations have begun to implement
the agreement.

The Gothenburg Protocol

Such problems were the target of the UNECE when it met in December 1999 in Gothenburg, Sweden, to sign its new agreement for controlling emissions of SO_2, NO_x, ammonia, and VOCs. Under the Gothenburg Protocol to Abate Acidification, Eutrophication, and Ground-Level Ozone, 27 nations (including the United States and Canada) agreed that international transport of these pollutants is significant enough to warrant international action. The European parties to this accord went a step further by agreeing that new emissions reductions should be mandated in the agreement based on the levels necessary to protect human health and ecosystems in specific downwind areas. That presents a departure from other international agreements, which have been based on countries' reducing emissions by a percentage that they deem economically or technically feasible.

But the accord is unique in other ways, too. "It's really a very important agreement in the field of international environmental policy making for several reasons," says Wuester. One reason is that the agreement involves many nations and covers a very wide geographic area including—despite the UNECE's name—Canada and the United States. Since Russia is also one of the 55 UNECE member states, agreements formed within this body have the potential to effect the vast majority of the Northern Hemisphere.

The Gothenburg Protocol—which [as of November 2003] has not been signed by Russia, Ukraine . . . or several other important polluters— is the eighth addition to the UNECE's Convention on Long-Range Transboundary Air Pollution, which was originally signed in 1979. Together, these protocols represent the world's largest international set of agreements on transported air pollutants to date. UNECE nations have agreed to limits on SO_2 (1987, 1994, 1999), NO_x (1991, 1999), VOCs (1997, 1999), heavy metals (1998), POPs (1998), and ammonia (1999). The framework convention to these agreements was signed by 44 nations.

According to the World Health Organization (WHO), air pollution causes 2.7 million deaths per year.

The Gothenburg Protocol is unique among these and other agreements also because it includes limits on multiple pollutants that have multiple effects. It recognizes that different environmental problems can be interconnected. "There was a common feature to the issues treated in the modeling work for this protocol," says Wuester. "Either the pollutants were common to a problem or the effects were common to a pollutant."

Addressing ground-level ozone in the protocol meant limiting emissions of NO_x and VOCs, which react to form ozone in sunlight. But NO_x also contributes to eutrophication (uncontrolled growth of plankton or algae), so that problem is included as well. Including eutrophication in the agreement also meant limiting SO_2 emissions, which along with NO_x lead to acidification of soil and water. Ammonia is also included because it too can raise the pH of soil and water.

For each of these problems, critical load maps were drawn for the whole of Europe showing the maximum pollutant concentration that each area could tolerate before detrimental environmental effects would be seen. These were coupled with deposition maps showing how much pollution flows into each area and where it originates. Finally, the costs of abatement were included so that the least expensive solution could be found. . . .

The Gothenburg Protocol is unique among these and other agreements . . . because it includes limits on multiple pollutants that have multiple effects.

While the modeling work used in the Gothenburg Protocol has been praised for its completeness, it only applies to Europe. For other parties to the protocol, namely the United States and Canada, no single model has emerged for finding the most cost-effective way to protect ecosystems and human health. "There are similar models for North America, though I guess it's fair to say that Canadian and U.S. scientists have not come up with one single model that they agree on," says Wuester.

Across the pond

Since North American emissions reductions were not dictated by the model used for European countries, Canada and the United States have been left to decide for themselves what levels of reduction should be included for them in the Gothenburg Protocol. According to Draper, for Canada and the United States, the commitments in the latest protocol defer to ongoing negotiations between the two nations. These negotiations are called for by the Canada-U.S. Air Quality Agreement, which the two nations signed in 1991. While that agreement was conceived to control acid rain, it created a framework for addressing other air pollution problems as well. In April of 1997, President Bill Clinton and Canadian Prime Minister Jean Chrétien decided the scope of the agreement should be broadened to include tropospheric ozone and particulate matter. First on the agenda is ozone. Negotiations to control this pollutant are ongoing, and any agreement resulting from those talks will also be integrated into the Gothenburg Protocol. . . .

In stark contrast to the situation in Europe where Spain, for example, will actually be making emissions reductions to protect other nations such as France, neither the United States nor Canada will make reductions specifically to protect the other. "We are not going to claim that we'll do more in the United States to help Canada than we would be doing anyway to help ourselves," says John Bachmann, the associate director for science/policy and new programs in the EPA's Office of Air Quality Planning and Standards, "but hopefully with this agreement we'll achieve some harmonization in the transboundary region."

So, while the Gothenburg Protocol will be a legally binding treaty with new emissions reductions for the nations of Europe, it will not be for the United States. "For us, this is an executive agreement," Bachmann says. "We can go up to and including things that are already mandated by our law. We can't go beyond that. Otherwise, we'd have to go to Congress to get it approved, and then it's no longer an executive agreement, it's a treaty. We're not doing a treaty here.". . .

But that does not mean that the North American countries have rejected the European loads-based approach outright. Bachmann says that some elements of a critical loads approach are integrated in the U.S. regional haze program as well as some water quality initiatives. "In Canada," says Draper, "we're homing in on the geographic source region that really needs to be controlled to move us most effectively toward looking at critical loads. I think there's a movement in both the United States and Canada to start to look at a much more integrated, comprehensive approach on air quality management, with a multipollutants and multieffects strategy."

The world versus POPs

New research is showing that some pollutants, including POPs, are carried much farther than previously thought. "There's been a fair amount of work done in North America, for example," says Buccini, "that shows when they're tilling the fields in the cotton-growing region of the southern United States—[in places] where they used toxaphene [a pesticide now classified as a POP] for many years—within three or four days you'll get spikes of toxaphene in rather predictable areas of the northern United States and Canada."

Also, POPs can be deposited in one country and then taken into another by air, water, or animals that ingest them. Wuester says this "grasshopper effect" makes it difficult to integrate POPs transport into the type of model on which the Gothenburg Protocol was based.

In North America, the U.S.-Canadian Great Lakes Water Quality Agreement has addressed POPs on a small regional level for over 25 years, while UNECE nations signed an agreement on them in 1998 that has not yet gone into force. Other bilateral and regional conventions exist as well. However, many feel an even broader agreement on POPs is needed. At a January–February 1997 meeting in Nairobi, Kenya, the UNEP Governing Council concluded that "a global, legally binding instrument is required to reduce the risks to human health and the environment [posed by POPs]."[2] . . .

"People are saying the nature of the problem may vary from country to country or region to region, but there is a basis here for taking global action."

"People are saying the nature of the problem may vary from country to country or region to region, but there is a basis here for taking global action," says Buccini. "There are 36 countries that are part of the [UN]ECE [protocol on POPs], but there's somewhere around 115 or 120 countries that are participating in the [UNEP] negotiations. For a lot of countries

2. In May 2001 the Stockholm Agreement on Persistent Organic Pollutants was signed.

there is no existing agreement." Thus, says Buccini, UNEP has an opportunity to drastically reduce worldwide emissions of POPs into the environment. If most of the countries involved in the negotiations ratify the agreement, the UNEP POPs convention could become the first truly global accord to address air pollutants that are deposited across boundaries.

The ultimate goal, says UNEP, is to eliminate all discharges, emissions, and losses of POPs around the world. On its "most wanted" list so far are 10 intentionally manufactured chemicals plus dioxins and furans, which are released chiefly as by-products of waste incineration. The 10 manufactured POPs, for the most part pesticides, include DDT and polychlorinated biphenyls. "With the exception of DDT, I think we are going to see . . . cessation of production," says Buccini. Countries that depend on DDT for controlling disease vectors such as mosquitoes that carry malaria will likely be allowed to continue limited use under the convention, he says.

The 1998 UNECE POPs agreement, which covers 16 substances, will be used as a stepping stone to the UNEP agreement. "Those countries within the UNECE that are parties to the POPs protocol will be trying to reflect their commitments under that protocol in the global instrument," says Buccini.

Emulating Europe

The European lead is being followed elsewhere as well. The World Bank is funding modeling work for air pollution transport in Asia that emulates the RAINS model used for the Gothenburg Protocol. Simultaneously, UNEP is collaborating with the Association of South East Asian Nations to fight the transport of haze from forest fires to nearby nations.

There are other efforts under way to protect nations from each other's air pollution. In North America, a trilateral agreement on air pollution is being formed under the auspices of the North American Free Trade Agreement. Regional agreements that protect the Great Lakes and the Georgia Basin ecosystem of southwest British Columbia and northwest Washington State have also been signed. In Europe, there are agreements to protect the Mediterranean and North Seas.

In addition to these are a smattering of local initiatives—agreements formed between towns or regions across the border from one another. For example, residents of Sault Sainte Marie, Michigan, were assisted by the EPA [Environmental Protection Agency] in reducing the emissions from a steel mill across the Canadian border. "We've had some real success with these initiatives at the city and county level," says Stephen Rothblatt, chief of the Air Programs Branch for EPA Region 5.

"In some locations we've got a whole bunch of different programs working at once," says Coronado. "The problem with this system is that you have all these pieces, and the question becomes where do they all fit. It's really hard to know. . . . People don't really know where to look when they are facing these issues." And besides creating unnecessary confusion, redundancy and waste in these programs is likely as well, he says.

"What we're working toward is to be able to look at transboundary air problems in a borderless context," says Draper. Research is constantly suggesting that such an approach is necessary. For example, metals transport from warm to cool climates is suggested as an explanation for why 83% of Inuit men and 73% of Inuit women in the eastern Canadian Arctic were found to have daily intakes of mercury above WHO guidelines, according to research by scientists from McGill University in Québec, Canada, published in the March 1997 issue of *EHP*. The UNECE adopted a protocol on heavy metals at the same time it adopted its POPs protocol, and Buccini sees it as likely that UNEP may follow suit.

Although recent UNECE protocols are being lauded and imitated, Wuester cautions that they are still largely untested. "Only the implementation itself will show us how important the agreements are for the environment," he says.

Organizations to Contact

The editors have compiled the following list of organizations concerned with the issues debated in this book. The descriptions are derived from materials provided by the organizations. All have publications or information available for interested readers. The list was compiled on the date of publication of the present volume; names, addresses, phone and fax numbers, and e-mail addresses may change. Be aware that many organizations take several weeks or longer to respond to inquiries, so allow as much time as possible.

American Council on Science and Health (ACSH)
1995 Broadway, 2nd Floor, New York, NY 10023-5860
(212) 362-7044 • fax: (212) 362-4919
e-mail: acsh@acsh.org • Web site: www.acsh.org

ACSH is a consumer education consortium concerned with, among other topics, issues related to the environment and health. The council publishes the quarterly *Priorities* magazine and position papers such as "Global Climate Change and Human Health" and "Corporate Greed or Children's Health?"

American Lung Association
61 Broadway, 6th Floor, New York 10006
(212) 315-8700
Web site: www.lungusa.org

The American Lung Association is a voluntary health organization dedicated to fighting lung disease in all its forms. It publishes numerous newsletters and papers dealing with lung health, including "The Weekly Breather" and *Asthma Magazine.*

Canadian Centre for Pollution Prevention (C2P2)
100 Charlotte St., Sarnia, ON N7T 4R2 Canada
(800) 667-9790 • fax: (519) 337-3486
e-mail: info@c2p2online.com • Web site: www.c2p2online.com

The Canadian Centre for Pollution Prevention is a nonprofit pollution prevention resource. It offers easy access to national and international information on air pollution and prevention through a search service, hard copy distribution, an extensive Web site, online forums, publications, and customized training. Among its publications are the *Practical Pollution Training Guide* and *At the Source*, C2P2's newsletter published three times a year.

Cato Institute
1000 Massachusetts Ave. NW, Washington, DC 20001-5403
(202) 842-0200 • fax (202) 842-3490
e-mail: cato@cato.org • Web site: www.cato.org

The Cato Institute is a libertarian public policy research foundation dedicated to limiting the role of government and protecting civil liberties. It disapproves of Environmental Protection Agency regulations, considering them too stringent. The institute publishes the quarterly magazine *Regulation*, the bimonthly

Cato Policy Report, and numerous papers dealing with air pollution, including "Why States, Not EPA, Should Set Pollution Standards" and "The EPA's Clean Air-ogance."

Clean Air Task Force (CATF)
77 Summer St., 8th Floor, Boston, MA 02110
(617) 292-0234
e-mail: info@catf.us • Web site: www.catf.us

CATF is a nonprofit organization dedicated to restoring clean air and a healthy environment through scientific research, public education, and legal advocacy. It publishes fact sheets and reports about air pollution, including "Children at Risk" and "Death, Disease, and Dirty Power."

Environmental Defense Fund (EDF)
257 Park Ave. S., New York 10010
(800) 684-3322 • fax: (212) 505-2375
e-mail: members@environmentaldefense.org • Web site: www.edf.org

EDF is a leading national nonprofit organization representing more than three hundred thousand members. It attempts to link science, economics, and law to cost-effective solutions to environmental problems. The organization is dedicated to protecting the environmental rights of all people, including access to clean air.

Environmental Protection Agency (EPA)
Ariel Ross Building, 1200 Pennsylvania Ave. NW, Washington, DC 20460
(202) 272-0167
e-mail: public-access@epa.gov • Web site: www.epa.gov

The EPA is the federal agency in charge of protecting the environment and controlling pollution. The agency works toward these goals by assisting businesses and local environmental agencies, enacting and enforcing regulations, identifying and fining polluters, and cleaning up polluted sites. It publishes the monthly *EPA Activities Update* and numerous periodic reports.

Environment Canada
351 St. Joseph Blvd., Gatineau, QC K1A 0H3 Canada
(819) 997-2800 • fax: (819) 953-2225
e-mail: enviroinfo@ec.gc.ca • Web site: www.ec.gc.ca

Environment Canada is a department of the Canadian government dedicated to achieving sustainable development in Canada through environmental protection and conservation. It publishes reports and fact sheets on a variety of environmental issues, including air pollution and climate change.

Foundation for Clean Air Progress (FCAP)
1801 K St. NW, Suite 1000L, Washington, DC 20036
(800) 272-1604
e-mail: info@cleanairprogress.org • Web site: www.cleanairprogress.org

FCAP is a nonprofit organization that believes that the public remains unaware of the substantial progress that has been made in reducing air pollution. It represents various sectors of business and industry in providing information to the public about improving air quality trends. In support of its call for less government regulation, FCAP publishes numerous studies and reports demonstrating that air pollution is on the decline.

Friends of the Earth
1025 Vermont Ave. NW, Washington, DC 20005-6303
(202) 783-7400 • fax: (202) 783-0444
e-mail: foe@foe.org • Web site: www.foe.org

Friends of the Earth is a national advocacy organization dedicated to the protection of the planet for future generations. It publishes the quarterly *Friends of the Earth* newsmagazine and *Atmosphere*, a report focusing on actions taken to preserve the ozone layer.

Heritage Foundation
214 Massachusetts Ave. NE, Washington, DC 20002-4999
(800) 546-2843 • fax: (202) 546-8328
e-mail: pubs@heritage.org • Web site: www.heritage.org

The Heritage Foundation is a conservative think tank that supports free enterprise and limited government. Its researchers criticize EPA overregulation. The foundation's publications, such as the quarterly *Policy Review*, include studies on the effectiveness of air pollution regulation.

INFORM
120 Wall St., New York, NY 10005-4001
(212) 361-2400 • fax: (212) 361-2412
e-mail: brown@informinc.org • Web site: www.informinc.org

INFORM is an independent research organization that examines the effects of business practices on the environment and on human health. The collective goal of its members is to identify ways of doing business that ensure environmentally sustainable economic growth. It publishes the quarterly newsletter *INFORM Reports* and fact sheets and reports on how to protect our natural resources and safeguard public health.

Reason Foundation
3415 S. Sepulveda Blvd., Suite 400, Los Angeles, CA 90034
(310) 391-2245 • fax: (310) 391-4395
e-mail: gpassantino@reason.org • Web site: www.reason.org

The foundation promotes individual freedoms and free-market principles. Its researchers believe that air quality is improving, and that the dangers of ozone depletion and global warming are myths. It publishes the monthly magazine *Reason*.

Sierra Club
85 Second St., 2nd Floor, San Francisco, CA 94105-3441
(415) 977-5500 • fax: (415) 977-5799
e-mail: information@sierraclub.org • Web site: www.sierraclub.org

The Sierra Club is a grassroots organization with chapters in every state. It promotes the protection and conservation of natural resources. In addition to books and fact sheets, it publishes the bimonthly magazine *Sierra* and the *Planet* newsletter, which appears several times a year.

World Resources Institute (WRI)
10 G St. NE, Suite 800, Washington, DC 20002
(202) 729-7600 • fax: (202) 729-7610
e-mail: lauralee@wri.org • Web site: www.wri.org

WRI provides information, ideas, and solutions to global environmental problems. Its mission is to encourage society to live in ways that protect Earth's environment for current and future generations. The institute's program attempts to meet global challenges by using knowledge to catalyze public and private action. WRI publishes the reports *Climate, Biodiversity, and Forests: Issues and Opportunities Emerging from the Kyoto Protocol* and *Climate Protection Policies: Can We Afford to Delay?*

Worldwatch Institute
1766 Massachusetts Ave. NW, Washington, DC 20036-1904
(202) 452-1999 • fax: (202) 296-7365
e-mail: worldwatch@worldwatch.org • Web site: www.worldwatch.org

Worldwatch is a nonprofit public policy research organization dedicated to informing policy makers and the public about emerging global problems and trends. It publishes the bimonthly *World Watch* magazine and several policy papers.

Web Site

Clean Air Now
Web site: www.cleanairnow.org

Clean Air Now is an alliance of citizen-funded public interest advocacy organizations that aims to protect public health from air pollution through informed action. It publishes numerous reports on air pollution, including *Danger in the Air: Unhealthy Levels of Smog in 2003,* and *Darkening Skies: Trends Toward Increasing Power Plant Emissions.*

Bibliography

Books

Pamela S. Chasek, ed. *The Global Environment in the Twenty-First Century: Prospects for International Cooperation.* Tokyo: United Nations University Press, 2000.

Judith A. Cherni *Economic Growth Versus the Environment: The Politics of Wealth, Health, and Air Pollution.* New York: Palgrave, 2002.

Robert G. Darst *Smokestack Diplomacy: Cooperation and Conflict in East-West Environmental Politics.* Cambridge, MA: MIT, 2001.

Terry Dinan and Christian Spoor *An Evaluation of Cap-and-Trade Programs for Reducing U.S. Carbon Emissions.* Washington, DC: Congress of the United States, Congressional Budget Office, 2001.

Francis Drake *Global Warming: The Science of Climate Change.* New York: Oxford University Press, 2000.

Indur Goklany *Clearing the Air: The Real Story of the War on Air Pollution.* Washington, DC: Cato Institute, 1999.

Hugh S. Gorman *Redefining Efficiency: Pollution Concerns, Regulatory Mechanisms, and Technological Changes in the U.S. Petroleum Industry.* Akron, OH: University of Akron Press, 2001.

Wyn Grant, Anthony Perl, and Peter Knoepfel, eds. *The Politics of Improving Urban Air Quality.* Northampton, MA: Edward Elgar, 1999.

S.T. Holgate et al., eds. *Air Pollution and Health.* London: Academic Press, 1999.

Jane Q. Koenig *Health Effects of Ambient Air Pollution: How Safe Is the Air We Breathe?* Boston: Kluwer Academic, 2000.

Gordon McGranahan and Frank Murray, eds. *Air Pollution and Health in Rapidly Developing Countries.* Sterling, VA: Earthscan, 2003.

Patrick J. Michaels and Robert Balling Jr. *The Satanic Gases: Clearing the Air About Global Warming.* Washington, DC: Cato Institute, 2000.

National Assessment Synthesis Team *Climate Change Impacts on the United States: The Potential Consequences of Climate Variability and Change.* Washington, DC: U.S. Global Change Research Program, 2000.

Gunter Pauli *Upsizing: The Road to Zero Emissions, More Jobs, More Income, and No Pollution.* Sheffield, England: Greenleaf, 2000.

David Wheeler *Racing to the Bottom? Foreign Investment and Air Pollution in Developing Countries.* Washington, DC: World Bank, Development Research Group, Infrastructure and Environment, 2001.

89

Periodicals

Martin Beniston	"Climactic Change: Possible Impacts on Human Health," *Swiss Medical Weekly*, 2002.
Katherine Bolt et al.	"Minute Particles, Major Problems: New Policies Show Promise for Saving Millions of Lives by Clearing the Air in the Developing World," *Forum for Applied Research and Public Policy*, Fall 2001.
Bert Brunekreef and Stephen T. Hotgate	"Air Pollution and Health," *Lancet*, October 2002.
Peter Burney	"Air Pollution and Asthma: The Dog That Doesn't Always Bark," *Lancet*, March 1999.
Marla Cone	"Vehicles Blamed for a Greater Share of Smog," *Los Angeles Times*, October 30, 1999.
Paula Court	"Do You Jog in Smog? Air Pollution Is Another Factor to Consider in Your Fitness Program," *American Fitness*, May/June 2002.
Jane K. Dixon	"Kids Need Clean Air: Air Pollution and Children's Health," *Family Community Health*, January 2002.
Gregg Easterbrook	"Environmental Doomsday: Bad News Good, Good News Bad," *Brookings Review*, Spring 2002.
A. Denny Ellerman and Paul L. Joskow	"Clearing the Polluted Sky," *New York Times*, May 1, 2001.
Foundation for Clean Air Progress	"Air Pollution Plummets as Energy Use Climbs," January 2002. www.cleanairprogress.org.
Issues and Controversies On File	"Air Pollution," March 1999.
Matthew E. Kahn	"The Beneficiaries of Clean Air Act Regulation," *Regulation*, Spring 2003.
Ben Lieberman	"The Counterproductive Clean Air Act," *CEI Update*, March 2000.
Randall Lutter	"Clean Air and Dirty Science," *Washington Times*, March 25, 2002.
Atrick J. Michaels	"Global Warming Warnings: A Lot of Hot Air," *USA Today Magazine*, January 2001.
Benoit Nemery, Peter H.M. Hoet, and Abderrahim Nemmar	"The Meuse Valley Fog of 1930: An Air Pollution Disaster," *Lancet*, March 2001.
Charles W. Petit	"A Darkening Sky (Effects of Pollution over Asia)," *U.S. News & World Report*, March 17, 2003.
Eric Pianin	"Study Ties Pollution, Risk of Lung Cancer Effects Similar to Secondhand Smoke," *Washington Post*, March 6, 2002.
Gary Polakovic	"Smog Feared in Power Buildup," *Los Angeles Times*, July 16, 2001.

Janet Raloff · "Air Sickness: How Microscopic Dust Particles Cause Subtle but Serious Harm," *Science News*, August 2003.

Jonathan Rauch · "America Celebrates Earth Day 1970—for the 31st Time," *Reason Online*, April 29, 2000. www.reason.com.

Andrew C. Revkin · "Record Ozone Hole Fuels Debate on Climate," *New York Times*, October 10, 2000.

Joel Schwartz · "Air Scare: Does Air Pollution Cause Asthma?" February 20, 2002. www.rppi.org.

Joel Schwartz · "Grading the Graders: How Advocacy Groups' 'Report Cards' Mislead the Public on Air Pollution and Urban Transport," December 2001. www.rppi.org.

Katharine Q. Seelye · "Study Sees 6,000 Deaths from Power Plants," *New York Times*, April 18, 2002.

UC Berkeley Wellness Letter · "The Great Indoors," February 1999.

U.S. Environmental Protection Agency · "Smog: Who Does It Hurt?: What You Need to Know About Ozone and Your Health," July 1999. www.epa.gov.

Christina Ward · "U.S. Unprepared for Global Warming's Health Effects," June 2001. www.disasterrelief.org.

Index

acid rain, 30
Acid Rain Program, 30
air pollutants
  asbestos, 17–18, 63
  biological, 18, 61–62
  carbon monoxide, 14, 29, 34, 57–58
  combustion by-products, 17
  house dust, 62–63
  lead, 13, 15, 29–30, 63
  major, 7, 13
  motor vehicle emissions, 14, 23, 29
  nitrogen oxides, 14, 15, 26–27, 34
  ozone, 13, 21, 22, 27–28, 34, 39–40
  particulate matter, 13–14, 21, 22,
    28–29, 34
  programs to reduce, 31–32
  radon, 18, 63, 64
  reductions in, 34–35
  sulfur dioxide, 14, 28, 34
  tobacco smoke, 16–18
  volatile organic compounds, 17, 57,
    60–61, 64
air pollution
  in Asia, 66–69
  death toll from, 7–8
  from diesel engines, 22
  global approach to, is necessary, 78
  global warming caused by
    will harm human health, 43–48
      con, 49–55
  international agreements to control,
    15–16
  is declining, 38–39
  misperceptions about, 35–36
  perception vs. reality of, 34–35
  from power plants, 21–22
  prevalence of, 37–38
  regional, 15
  threatens human health, 20–24
  threat from, is exaggerated, 33–42
  see also indoor air pollution;
    outdoor air pollution
Air Pollution Control Act (1955), 12
air quality
  Americans' perceptions about, 35–36
  has improved, 7–8, 19, 25–32, 41
  is not up to standards, 23–24
  monitoring of, 7

regulation reforms
  will improve, 75–77
  will worsen, 70–74
air toxins, 30–32
  see also air pollutants
American Council on Science and
  Health (ACSH), 50–51
American Lung Association, 7, 9, 36,
  37–39, 40
asbestos, 17–18, 63
Asia, 66–69
automobile emissions, 14, 23, 29,
  38–39

Bachmann, John, 81–82
benzene, 31
Bond, Christopher, 75
Bower, John, 56
Brookings Institution, 8
Buccini, John, 79, 82, 84
Bush, George W., 9

Calderera, Michael, 59
Canada-U.S. Air Quality Agreement
  (1991), 81
cancer, 23
carbon monoxide, 14, 29, 34, 57–58
children, 19
China
  air quality in, 8, 67–68
  changing weather patterns in, 69
chlorination by-products, 60–61
Clean Air Act (1970), 7, 12
  criticisms of, 8–9
  EPA responsibilities under, 26
  New Source Review provisions, 9,
    70–77
  reforms of
    will improve air quality, 75–77
    will worsen air quality, 70–74
Clean Air Act Amendments (1990), 15
climate change. See global warming
Clinton, Bill, 49
combustion by-products, 17

deaths
  from air pollution, 7–8, 79
  heat-related, 44–45

in winter vs. summer, 54
diesel engines, 22, 35
diseases, 52–53
Donora catastrophe, 7, 12
drought, 46
dust, 62–63
dust mites, 61–62, 64

Earth Policy Institute, 7
Easterbrook, Gregg, 8
Edwards, John, 70
El Niño, 47, 67, 69
environmentalists, exaggerated claims
  by, 33, 36–42
Environmental Protection Agency
  (EPA), 7
  air quality standards set by, 25
  critics of, 8–9
  emissions standards of, 31–32
  ozone monitoring by, 34
  responsibilities of, under Clean Air
    Act, 26
  role of, 12–13

Fischlowitz-Roberts, Bernie, 7–8
flooding, 46
formaldehyde, 17, 60
fossil fuels, 12, 17
Franke, Deborah, 65

gas heaters, 57, 58–60, 64
gas stoves, 59–60, 64
global warming
  benefits of, 55
  hotspots, 44–47
  recent and projected, 44
  will harm human health, 43–48
    con, 49–55
Gore, Al, 49–50
Gothenburg Protocol, 80–81
greenhouse gases, 48
  see also global warming
Greiner, Thomas, 59

hazardous air pollutants (HAPs),
  22–23
health effects
  of air pollution, 7–8, 11–24
  of asbestos, 17–18
  of biologic contaminants, 18
  of carbon monoxide, 14, 57–58
  of combustion by-products, 17
  of global warming
    will be harmful, 43–48
      con, 49–55
  of indoor air pollution, 56–65

of nitrogen dioxide, 14
of ozone, 13, 21, 39–40
of particulate matter, 13–14, 21
of population growth, 51
of radon, 18
of sulfur dioxide, 14
of tobacco smoke, 17
of volatile organic compounds, 17
Healthy People 2000, 19
heart disease, 12
heat waves, 44–45
Homa, David, 11
housecleaning methods, 65
hurricanes, 54–55
hydrochloric acid, 21–22

India, 68
indoor air pollution
  is major health risk, 56–65
  reducing, 18, 63–65
  sources of, 16–18, 57–65
infectious diseases, 52–53
international pollution agreements,
  78–84

Jacobson, Mark, 69

Kiehl, Jeff, 68
Kirkwood, John, 9
Kovats, R. Sari, 43
Kyoto protocol, 49

lead, 13, 15, 29–30, 63
Lewis, Robert G., 62–63
London, England, 12
lung disease, 12, 13, 17–18

malaria, 47, 52, 53
malnutrition, 46, 51–52
Mannino, David, 11
Manuel, John, 56
Marksen, Craig S., 8–9
Maximum Achievable Control
  Technology (MACT), 23
Menon, Surabi, 69
mercury, 22
molds, 61–62, 64
Moore, Thomas Gale, 49
Motor Vehicle Air Pollution Act
  (1965), 12
motor vehicle emissions, 14, 23, 29,
  38–39
Myer, Pamela, 11

Naeher, Luke, 11
National Ambient Air Quality

Standards (NAAQS), 7, 20
National-Scale Air Toxins Assessment
    (NATA), 23
New Source Review (NSR) provisions, 9
    will improve air quality, 75–77
    will worsen air quality, 70–74
nitrogen oxides, 14, 15, 26–27, 34
nonroad heavy-duty diesel engines
    (HDDEs), 22
North American Free Trade
    Agreement (NAFTA), 16
Northeast Ozone Transport Region, 15

outdoor air pollution
    causes of, 12–14
    controlling, 14–16
    spread of, 15
ozone, 13, 21, 22, 27–28, 34, 36–40
Ozone Transport Assessment Group
    (OTAG), 15

parasitic diseases, 52–53
particulate matter (PM), 13–14, 21,
    22, 28–29, 34
Patz, Jonathan A., 43
Petit, Charles W., 66
polybrominated duphenyl ethers
    (PBDEs), 61
power plants, 21–22
Public Interest Research Group
    (PIRG), 36, 38, 40, 50

radon, 18, 63, 64
Raloff, Janet, 8
Redd, Stephen, 11
regulations
    changes in, under Bush
        administration, 9, 70–77
    criticisms of, 8–9
    debate over, 7
    global approach to, is necessary,
        78–84
    international agreements, 15–16,
        78–84

Motor Vehicle Air Pollution Act, 12
    reforms of
        will improve air quality, 75–77
        will worsen air quality, 70–74
    see also Clean Air Act
Reuther, Christopher G., 78
Rosenfeld, Daniel, 68

Schwartz, Joel, 33
sea level rise, 45
Sierra Club, 39, 50
Southern Appalachian Mountains
    Initiative, 15
sport-utility vehicles (SUVs), 38–39
sulfur dioxide, 14, 28, 34

tetraethyl lead, 13
tobacco smoke, 16, 17, 18
tornadoes, 54–55
tropical diseases, 52–53

United Nations Economic
    Commission for Europe (UNECE),
    79–80
United Nations Environment
    Programme (UNEP), 78–84
United States
    global regulations on air pollution
        and, 78–84
    pollution-associated health
        problems in, 8
    production of greenhouse gases by,
        48
utilities, electric, 21–22

volatile organic compounds (VOCs),
    17, 57, 60–61, 64

Weisel, Clifford, 60–61
Williams, Arthur L., 20
World Health Organization (WHO),
    51, 79
Wuester, Henning, 79–81